Ultrasonography in Obstetrics and Gynecology

second edition

Ultrasonography in Obstetrics and Gynecology

second edition

John C. Hobbins, M.D.
Professor
Department of Obstetrics and Gynecology and Diagnostic Radiology
Yale University School of Medicine
Director of Obstetrics
Yale-New Haven Hospital
New Haven, Connecticut

Fred Winsberg, M.D.
Professor of Radiology
McGill University, Faculty of Medicine
Diagnostic Radiologist-in-Chief
Montreal General Hospital
Quebec, Canada

Richard L. Berkowitz, M.D.
Professor
Department of Obstetrics and Gynecology
Mt. Sinai School of Medicine
Director, Division of Maternal-Fetal Medicine
Mt. Sinai Medical Center
New York, New York

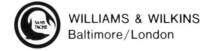

WILLIAMS & WILKINS
Baltimore/London

Copyright ©, 1983
Williams & Wilkins
428 East Preston Street
Baltimore, MD 21202, U.S.A.

Made in the United States of America

First edition 1977
    Reprinted 1978, 1980, 1981
Second Edition, 1983
    Reprinted 1984

Library of Congress in Publication Data

Main entry under title:

Ultrasonography in obstetrics and gynecology.

    Includes index.
    1. Ultrasonics in obstetrics. 2. Generative organs, Female—Diseases—Diagnosis. 3. Diagnosis, Ultrasonic. I. Hobbins, John C. II. Winsberg, Fred. III. Berkowitz, Richard L. [DNLM: 1. Fetal diseases—Diagnosis. 2. Genital diseases, Female—Diagnosis. 3. Obstetrics. 4. Ultrasonics—Diagnostic Use. WQ 240 H682u]
RG527.5.U48U47 1983   618.2′07543   82-11185
ISBN 0-683-04089-8

Composed and printed at the
Waverly Press, Inc.
Mt. Royal and Guilford Aves.
Baltimore, MD 21202, U.S.A.

Preface to the Second Edition

Since the first edition of this book the scope of obstetrical ultrasound has broadened appreciably and many initial concepts have been replaced by new ones. Not surprisingly, the impressive progress made in obstetrical ultrasound has been accompanied by growing pains imposed by our complex society. Ultrasound organizations have been wrestling with the delicate tasks of formulating minimum requirements of training and suggesting methods of certification. In addition, because of pressures from third party payers and interdepartmental politics, there has been a demand for clarification concerning the issue of who should scan the obstetrical and gynecological patient.

The concept of Stage I and Stage II ultrasound examinations emanated from protocols designed for maternal serum alphafetoprotein (MSAFP) screening. Here ultrasound would be used in two distinctly different ways: 1. To rule out obvious reasons for high MSAFP levels such as wrong dates, intrauterine demise, or multiple gestation. 2. To identify the subtle spinal defect, ventral wall defect, or cystic hygroma in patients with high amniotic fluid levels of AFP. The frequently required Stage I examination could be performed by a trained ultrasound generalist and the Stage II examination, required in one or two of every 1,000 patients screened, could be performed by a specialist with significant experience in this type of demanding evaluation. Since this concept seemed to make sense, some have now advocated expanding it to include other types of obstetrical evaluations.

It is not within the design of this text to comment on the predominantly political issues of who should scan, how much training he or she should have, or whether the Stage I, Stage II concept should be expanded. Instead, the book is designed to provide a concise and straightforward approach to reams of complex and sometimes controversial data in the literature to which the busy ultrasound user is constantly exposed. As in the first edition, when dealing with unresolved issues we will inject our common opinion in an effort to provide the reader with a uniform approach to difficult subjects. It will be quite clear where these opinions appear. Also, no chapter in this edition has been written exclusively by one author, and each concept has been treated so that ultrasound findings are correlated with basic principles in fetal and maternal physiology.

The last chapter in the first edition was devoted to the gynecological examination. Our literature scan has not produced enough new information regarding ultrasound's efficiency in defining pelvic tumors to warrant a chapter on this subject. A new field, however, has recently emerged in which ultrasound plays an invaluable role—the treatment of the infertile patient. One can now closely observe with ultrasound the maturing follicle so that coitus or in vitro fertilization can be timed precisely. Also, the effects of ovulation-stimulating drugs can be serially assessed. Because of ultrasound's exciting role in these ventures, a chapter on the ovary has been added to the text.

The response to the first edition of this book has been extremely gratifying. We hope that the reader will find this new edition to be an equally practical review of the current state of the art in obstetrical ultrasound.

Acknowledgment

We are deeply indebted to Ingeborg Venus for her tireless efforts in editing manuscripts and coordinating in a tri-authored text. Without her invaluable effort this book would still be "in press".

Contents

Preface to the second edition   v

Acknowledgment   vii

Chapter 1
Brief introduction
to scanning   1

Chapter 2
Early pregnancy   13

Chapter 3
Estimation
of gestational age   34

Chapter 4
The placenta   46

Chapter 5
Third trimester
complications   62

Chapter 6
Intrauterine
growth retardation   87

Chapter 7
Normal & Abnormal
fetal anatomy   113

Chapter 8
Invasive Procedures   170

Chapter 9
Ultrasound evaluation
of fetal dynamics   203

Chapter 10   210
Ultrasound in
ovarian evaluation

Appendix   216

Index   237

Brief Introduction to Scanning

The aim of this section is not to provide an exhaustive discussion of the physical principles of ultrasound, but to deal with those problems which are currently of interest and which may be controversial. Although ultrasound is technically defined as sound of higher frequency than that which is audible to the human ear, in clinical practice it is limited to frequencies in the range from 1 to 10 million cycles/sec., that is, 1 to 10 MHz. Obstetrical ultrasound is performed in the range of 3 to 5 MHz, usually at 3.5 MHz and occasionally at 5 MHz. Although transmission methods of ultrasonic imaging have been developed, they have not proved to be of clinical value; current modes of examination employ reflected ultrasound, so-called echography. In this method, echoes returning from reflecting surfaces within the body are detected and analyzed. As the transmitted pulse from the transducer traverses the body, energy is reflected back to the transducer from organ interfaces, vessel walls, and parenchymal structure. The amount of energy reflected from organ interfaces depends upon the orientation of the reflecting interface and the difference in acoustic impedance of the tissues at the interface. The quantity of energy reaching a given organ or tissue interface is a function of the attenuation of the beam by the intervening tissue. The physical basis of parenchymal reflections from within organs such as the placenta and liver is not well understood, but they are probably the result of interfaces between marcromolecules of protein, water, and lipid. Ultrasonograms are the result of the interplay of *two* acoustic properties of tissue, reflection and attenuation. Each of these must be evaluated independently of the other in interpreting an ultrasonogram. A tissue may be both anechoic and attenuating or nonattenuating as well as reflecting. Tissues or masses may thus be described as echogenic vs. anechoic, sonolucent vs. attenuating, or any of the four possible combinations. With current systems the same transducer is used both for transmitting and receiving. This is possible because the duration of each pulse is small compared to the time between pulses. There are several methods of detecting and displaying the reflected echoes. These methods will be briefly reviewed. They include A-mode, B-mode, M-mode, and B-scanning.

In A-mode, or amplitude modulation, echoes are displayed as vertical spikes along the baseline of the cathode ray tube, with the height of the spike being related to the amplitude of the detected echo.

In B-mode, or brightness modulation, instead of being displayed as vertical spikes, the amplitude is represented by a spot of light on the cathode ray tube, the brightness of which is related to the intensity of the reflected echo. B-mode is used for two-dimensional scanning or echotomography (B-scanning) and is also used for time-motion studies (M-mode). The latter application is primarily in the field of pediatric and adult cardiology, but it is also of value in studying the fetal heart.

A-mode or amplitude modulation remains a valuable clinical tool in ultrasound. The dynamic range that one can display with A-mode is greater than that which can be displayed with intensity modulation, but the anatomical information provided by a single beam of sound is difficult to interpret and the amplitude varies drastically with the orientation of the reflecting surface to the sound beam. Current applications of A-mode include the aspiration transducer, a transducer with a central hole to localize fluid cavities and the position of an aspiration needle within them, and echocardiography, in which the anatomical structures being examined have characteristic motion patterns. It is useful to have A-mode available in conjunction with B-scanning. When the two methods are used simultaneously, the B-scan is the source of anatomical information whereas the A-mode representation may be used for a measurement of amplitude and distance.

There are various ways of producing B-scans. Until the past few years the most commonly used ultrasound machine in obstetrical practice was the articulated static scanner. An image is obtained by moving the transducer over the surface of the body and displaying the echoes in B-mode. The transducer arm has sensors, either analog or digital, at its joints that provide positional and directional information.

The operator of an articulated static B-scanner has considerable flexibility in the motions that he may use to examine the patient. A group of overlapping sectors or arcs may be put together to form a compound scan. This procedure has the advantage of providing a maximal amount of information about acoustic interfaces since the tissues are approached from a variety of angles. But compound scanning has several disadvantages:

1   The more complex the motion performed by the examiner, the longer is the time required to produce a scan, and motion produces distortion.
2   Valuable information about transmission and attenuation, such as acoustic shadowing and enhanced transmission through liquids, that is visible with simple scanning is obscured with compound scanning.
3   Artifacts can be introduced that depend upon the number of times a particular tissue is scanned, how long the transducer is held in a particular position, and other variables of operator technique.

The fundamental difficulty with B-scanning is that one is always dealing with a slice or tomogram. With manually operated equipment it is not feasible to produce every possible slice in every possible direction so as to reconstruct a three-dimensional picture of the relevant anatomy. The automated water path scanner of Kossoff (Ausonics Octoson) produces multiple tomographic sections in a relatively short time, but this instrument has several important disadvantages:

1   It is elaborate and expensive.
2   The patient must be examined prone.
3   The transducers are not in registration with each other so that a feathery tissue texture is obtained. Lack of registration probably arises from mechanical and acoustic factors. The latter includes failure to correct for refraction and unequal water path lengths resulting in slightly different average velocities of sound.

The fetus cannot be followed around readily, and even some standard sections such as the biparietal plane cannot be routinely obtained.

A selection of tomographic sections illustrating the anatomical and pathological features that the clinician wishes to see must somehow be culled from the infinite number of sections that is theoretically obtainable. How does one get around this problem?

"Real-time" ultrasonic tomography is certainly the best way to make an intelligent assessment of three-dimensional anatomy, observe moving structures, and properly select clinically useful anatomical cross sections. Articulated static scanning can be reserved for sections of the entire uterus to measure intrauterine volume or to image the entire placenta or fetus.

Articulated scanning remains the preferred method of providing a map for aspirations such as amniocentesis, unless specific real-time aspiration transducers are available. Real-time imaging has improved so dramatically in the last few years that any difference in image quality with the best real-time instruments is insignificant.

Current parlance distinguishes between real-time and B-scanning or gray scale. This distinction is incorrect since real-time scans are B-scans, that is they are two-dimensional B-mode images and they are intensity modulated and thus exhibit gray scale. In fact, early real-time images displayed gray scale before static images did because real-time images do not in principle require a storage scope. They are perceived as continuous if the frame rate exceeds flicker fusion frequency, whereas before the introduction of the analog scan converter in 1974, practically all static B-scans were recorded with bistable storage oscilloscopes. The production of gray scale images required prolonged exposure photography, a procedure most people doing ultrasonography long ago considered cumbersome. The real-time scanner provides x,y (position) and z (amplitude) axis acoustic data just as the static scanner. The spatial information provided by the static scanner is more complete, i.e., the position of the structures being imaged is determined with respect to the surface of the earth, whereas the real-time scanner relates the position of a structure only to the scanner. The static scanner can, in general, provide a larger field of view so that a global (CT like) image of the body can be made. *Neither the static nor the real-time scanner provides absolute positional information with respect to the body* except that which is derived from knowledge of anatomy, although some machines of each type are capable of indicating the position of a scan section relative to a section previously coded by the operator. Proponents of static scanners often misunderstand this limitation.

Although real-time systems do not require a storage scope at rapid frame rates, the digital memory (scan converter) has enhanced the usefulness of real-time instruments by adding the capability of high quality freeze-frames, frame rates lower than flicker fusion and even slow sweeps, and compatibility with television and multiformat cameras. The beam scanning mechanism determines the required capabilities of the scan converter. For example, a linear array requires a less sophisticated memory than a sector scanner. In the latter, ''holes'' in the image must be filled in by numerical manipulation as the lines of sight diverge from the transducer and the number of picture elements that need to be addressed increases with the square of the distance. With the marriage of scan converters to real-time, the speed of the memory as well as the finite velocity of sound (pixel acquisition time) is a limiting factor on frame rate and field size.

A useful classification of contemporary real-time scanners is into four basic categories:

1 Mechanical water path
   (a) Linear
   (b) Sector
2 Mechanical short fluid path
   (a) Rotating
   (b) Oscillating
3 Phased focused linear sequenced array
4 Steered array

The water path scanner

Water path scanners include a diverse group of beam scanning mechanisms that share one essential feature. The length of the water path between the transducer and the patient's skin is equal to the depth in the body one wishes to examine. Since the velocity of sound is finite at 1540 msec.$^{-1}$ for soft tissue

$$F \times N = \frac{77,000}{P + R} \text{ lines sec.}^{-1} \text{ sec.}^{-1}$$

where F is the number of frames sec.$^{-1}$;
       N is the number of ultrasound lines per frame;
       P is the penetration into the patient in centimeters plus equivalent distance in the imaging head fluid path;
       R is the recovery time expressed in centimeters of depth.
       (F $\times$ N is the pulse repetition frequency.)

For a water path system, "P" is slightly more than doubled since the velocity of sound in water is 1480 msec.$^{-1}$. One must, therefore, sacrifice one of three variables: frame rate, lines per frame, or depth. For abdominal systems, 20 cm of penetration are required and the number of lines per frame cannot be reduced without reducing the quality of the image so that frame rate and field size are sacrificed. Another problem encountered with water path systems is that the mass of water in the bath adds bulk and reduces maneuverability.

On the positive side of the balance sheet, a large transducer with a long focal length can be used so that lateral resolution is excellent (Figure 1).

Figure 1

Water path delay scanner utilizing dynamic focusing and oscillating mirror.

(Courtesy of Smith Kline Instruments.)

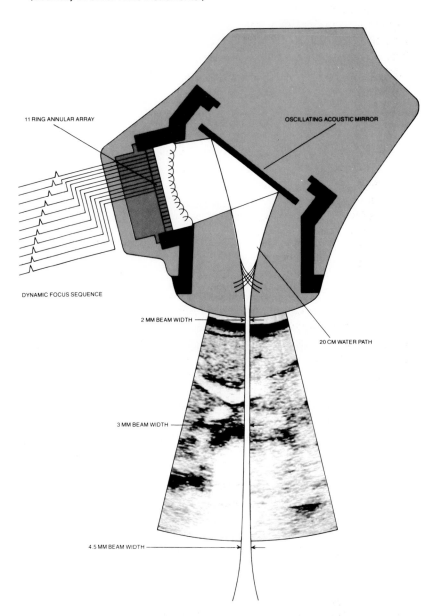

11 RING ANNULAR ARRAY

OSCILLATING ACOUSTIC MIRROR

DYNAMIC FOCUS SEQUENCE

2 MM BEAM WIDTH

20 CM WATER PATH

3 MM BEAM WIDTH

4.5 MM BEAM WIDTH

Short fluid path

In contrast to the water path scanner the short fluid path scanner uses a path length much less than the penetration in the body. The liquid attenuates the sound, particularly the higher frequency components, and refracts it. The degree of attenuation is a function of the fluid and membrane, and refraction occurs when the velocity of sound of the fluid is different from that of tissue. Since some systems use liquids of significantly lower acoustic velocity, such as mineral oil, refractive effects on beam focusing and image geometry must be considered. A liquid with velocity of sound less than tissue focuses the beam and diverges it from the perpendicular as the sound enters the body. Transducer rotation has theoretical advantages over oscillation since the angular velocity is constant, whereas with oscillation it is sinusoidal with a peak velocity in the center of the image.* Advantages of oscillation are:

1   By oscillating the transducer around its own axis one can obtain a large field of view for a small acoustic window, a factor that promotes good intercostal access.
2   Oscillation can provide higher frame rates since there is no dead time between transducer firings.
3   There are no transducer mating problems as only one transducer is employed.

The diameter of the transducer and the type of focusing are important determinants of resolution. Thirteen-millimeter transducer real-time devices are out of focus deeper than 10 cm but are suitable for more superficial structures. Nineteen-millimeter transducers provide improved depth resolution but require a larger surface of access for the head. At least three manufacturers (Diasonics, General Electric, and Phillips) incorporate low frequency filters that compensate for absorption of higher frequencies and improve the lateral resolution in depth.

Within the broad category of short fluid path scanners a variety of mechanisms for rotation and oscillation have been manufactured (Figure 2a and b). Some devices of this type use stationary or oscillating mirrors, and one device designed for simultaneous two-dimensional echocardiography and M-mode uses a beam-splitting mirror.

In the first generation mechanical sector scanners, the transducer oscillates or rotates in direct contact with the skin. These are rarely used for obstetrical applications. Although this method avoids some of the problems associated with selection of a liquid, it is stressful for the examiner, patient, and motor.

---

* It is possible to compensate for this anomaly of oscillation by varying the pulsing of the transducer to maintain a constant spatial frequency.

Figure 2

Oscillating mechanical sector scanner with short liquid path (usually castor oil). *b.* Rotating mechanical sector scanner.

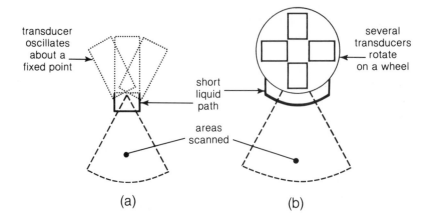

(a)   (b)

Focused linear array

The linear array first appeared on the market at about the same time as the analog scan converter. Lateral resolution was soon improved by dividing the transducer elements into subgroups and firing these subgroups or segments sequentially (Figure 3). Further improvement in geometry has been provided in the last 2 years by introducing firing delays within the subgroups of transducer elements such that the elements on the ends are fired before those in the middle (synthetic focus) (Figure 4). Receive focusing employing analogous receiver delays has also been incorporated (Figure 5). These timing maneuvers only affect the focus in the plane of the array. Focusing at right angles to the array is accomplished by mechanical means.

With refinements in firing sequence the resolution of linear arrays has improved dramatically, so that a wide variety of applications has developed, including obstetrical, abdominal, and small-parts imaging. The linear format is particularly suitable for fetal imaging, but the shape of the transducer head and swept beam limits subcostal examinations of the liver, kidney, examination of the pelvis, and sometimes the fundus or cervix of the gravid uterus. Linear arrays are probably the least trouble-prone devices we have in ultrasound. They are small, relatively portable, and rarely require the attention of a serviceman.

Both Kossoff in Australia and Pourcelot in France have developed steered linear arrays that can be operated in

Figure 3

Principle of segmented or co-phased linear array. Three successive pulses of four elements are shown (a, b, c,).

(From Wilkinson (10).)

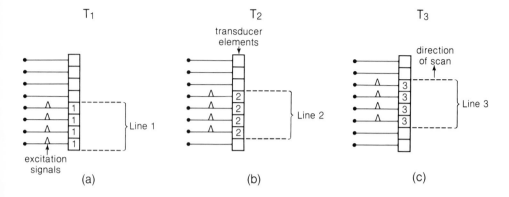

(a)   (b)   (c)

Figure 4

Transmit focusing. T_1, T_2, and T_3 are delay lines with T_3 representing the shortest and T_1 the longest delay.

(Modified from Wilkinson (10).)

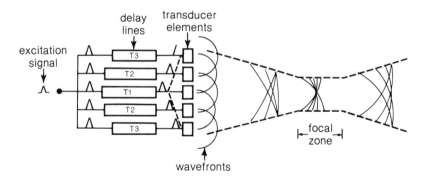

compound as well as linear mode, and curved arrays are being developed in Japan. These are not yet commercially available.

Phased arrays

The phased, or more properly, steered array is also made possible by time delay resulting in synthetic steering and transmit and receive focusing (Figure 6). Another term used to describe these devices is the electronic sector scanner to distinguish them from the

Figure 5

Receive focusing. T_1 is again the longest delay and T_3 the shortest.

(Modified from Wilkinson (10).)

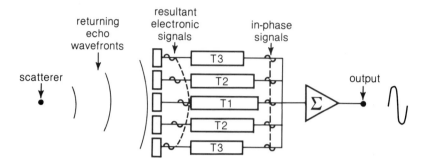

mechanical sector scanners described earlier. Phased arrays are rarely used in obstetrical imaging but may be particularly useful in guiding punctures, since a wide field of view is associated with a small window.

Real-time aspiration and puncture transducers

A linear array may be fitted with a slit so that needles can be advanced under real-time guidance. A mechanical sector scanner can be equipped with a laterally placed needle holder such that the needle will be advanced in a predictable and visible trajectory. Both of these devices have been produced in limited quantities but are not generally available commercially. The linear array aspiration transducers must be gas sterilized before each use, whereas the mechanical sector scanner can be enclosed in a sterile glove.

Summary of real-time devices

The linear array has become the workhorse of obstetrical ultrasound because of its low cost, portability, and shape. Mechanical sector scanners are more expensive but provide better resolution and access at somewhat lower frame rate. It is likely that both types of devices will be with us for the next 5 to 10 years. Better and cheaper steered arrays may also become interesting for obstetrics. There is only one water path real-time system now commercially available; it provides excellent image quality, but it is relatively expensive and less flexible than hand-held devices.

Measurements

Measurement errors with sonography are readily made if anatomical landmarks are not strictly reproduced. But

Figure 6

The use of variable delay lines to achieve beam steering.

(Modified from Wilkinson (10).)

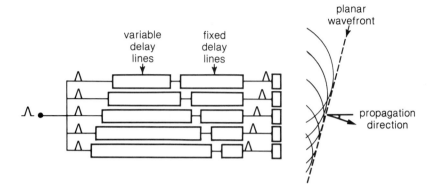

they also arise from physical limitations of the instruments. Axial resolution depends on pulse length, the product of wave length and wave number. For practical purposes this is no better than 1 mm at 3.5 MHz. Lateral resolution is a function of beam width and varies with depth and the diameter, frequency, and focusing of the transducer. It may be as large as 7 mm. Measurement is also affected by non-uniformity in tissue propagation velocity, the resolution and curvature of cathode ray tubes, and the accuracy of the mechanical or electronic calipers used to make the measurements.

A realistic attitude toward the biological, physical, instrumentational, and human limitations of measurements must be maintained. Anyone who claims he can measure a fetal head to within 0.5 mm is kidding himself no matter how elegant the statistical methods he uses and how impressive his results.

Suggested Readings

1   **Bom, N., Lancée, C.T., Honkoop, J., Hugenholtz, P.G.:** Ultrasonic viewer for cross-sectional analyses of moving cardiac structures. Biomed. Eng. 6:500, 1971.

2   **Bow, C.R., McDicken, W.N., Anderson, T., Scorgie, R.E., Muir, A.L.:** A rotating transducer real-time scanner for ultrasonic examination of the heart and abdomen. Br. J. Radiol. 52:29, 1979.

3   **Griffith, J.M., Henry, W.L.:** A sector scanner for real-time two-dimensional echocardiography. Circulation 49:1147, 1974.

4   **Holm, H.H., Kristensen, J.K., Pedersen, J.F., Hancke, S.,**

Northeved, A.: A new mechanical real-time ultrasonic contact scanner. Ultrasound Med. Biol. 2:19, 1975.

5   Kossoff, G.: Large waterpath ultrasonic scanners. Clin. Diagn. Ultrasound 5:85, 1980.

6   Krause, W., Soldner, R.: Ultrasonic imaging technique (B scan) with high image rate for medical diagnosis. Electromedica 4:8, 1967.

7   Skolnick, M.L., Matzuk, T.: A new ultrasonic real-time scanner featuring a servo-controlled transducer displaying a sector image. Radiology 128:439, 1978.

8   von Ramm, O.T., Thurstone, F.L.: Cardiac imaging using a phased array ultrasound system. I. System design. Circulation 53:258, 1976.

9   Wells, P.N.T.: Real-time scanning systems. Clin. Diagn. Ultrasound 5:69, 1980.

10   Wilkinson, R.W.: Principles of real-time two-dimensional B-scan ultrasonic imaging. J. Med. Eng. Technol. 5:21, 1981.

11   Winsberg, F.: Real-time scanners: A review. Med. Ultrasound 3:99, 1979.

Early Pregnancy

2

The best starting point for the discussion of early pregnancy is an examination of the non-pregnant uterus. It is generally recognized that an adequate ultrasonic examination of the uterus requires that the patient have a full bladder. Nonetheless, when a patient arrives without a full bladder, one is always tempted to conduct the examination in order to save time and spare the patient further inconvenience. This temptation should be resisted. The bladder must cover the fundus of the uterus. If the uterus tends to be anteverted, a full bladder will depress it and make its examination easier. If the uterus is retroverted, a full bladder will at least push bowel away from the fundus. Examining the patient who has an empty bladder will only lead to frustration and diagnostic errors. A too full bladder may displace a mass out of the pelvis and render it invisible (Figure 1). An overfilled bladder also elongates and flattens the uterus and has been blamed for false diagnoses of placenta previa and blighted ovum.

The widest anteroposterior portion of the bladder lies above the narrowest portion of the uterus, the cervix. As one moves superiorly, the bladder becomes narrower as the uterus becomes wider. A centrally located linear echo is observed in the uterus either at the level of the cervix or in the fundus. It represents the interface between adjacent levels of endometrium and is surrounded by a sonolucent halo of endometrium during the progestational phase.

Demonstration of a fundal cavity interface echo is an important clinical finding since it excludes the diagnosis of an intrauterine pregnancy (2). The cavity echo should not be mistaken for an intrauterine device (IUD). Intrauterine devices of various types are identified by their geometry and acoustic shadowing but the IUD must lie in the focused portion of the acoustic beam to produce an acoustic shadow. Often an IUD can be shown to contain both an entrance and exit reflection.

The diagnosis of pregnancy can be made about 5 to 6 weeks after the last menstrual period. A rounded fluid-containing sac is seen in the uterus which has been called the gestational sac (Figure 2). Embryologically, it

14

Figure 1

Sagittal scan of bladder. *a*. The bladder is overdistended and extends above the gravid uterus. *b*. After emptying of the bladder a cystic ovarian mass can be appreciated superior to the uterus.

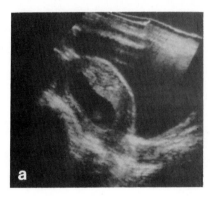
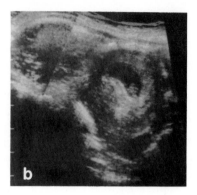

Figure 2

Gestational sac at 6 weeks and chorionic reaction around it. Fetal cardiac activity could not yet be appreciated.

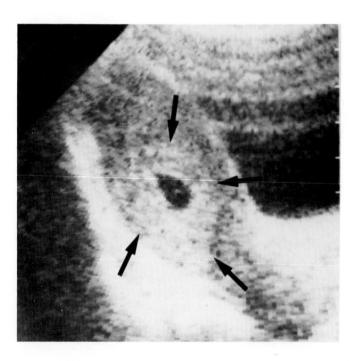

Figure 3

A. Illustration of components of early pregnancy. *B.* As pregnancy progresses placenta occupies a fundal position.

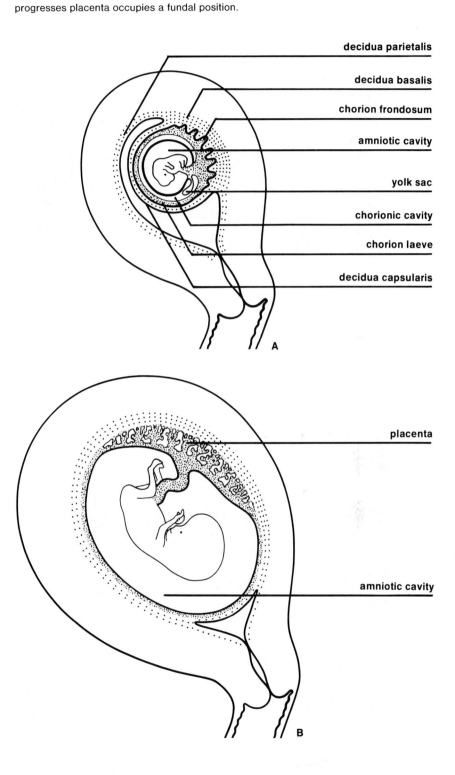

decidua parietalis

decidua basalis

chorion frondosum

amniotic cavity

yolk sac

chorionic cavity

chorion laeve

decidua capsularis

A

placenta

amniotic cavity

B

Figure 4

Seven-week gestation. The chorion frondosum (*lower black arrow*) is now distinguishable from the chorion laeve (*small arrows*). The embryo and fetal cardiac activity were seen (*large curved arrow*).

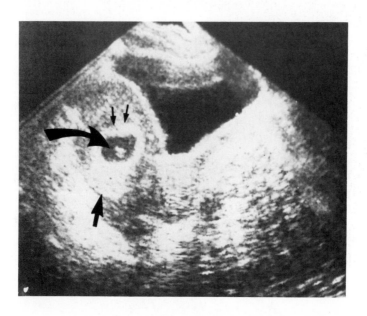

Figure 5

The fetus at 8 weeks with yolk sac visible.

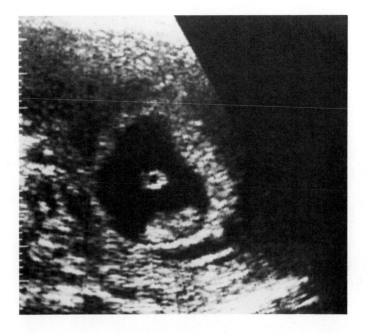

Figure 6

Incomplete fusion of amnion with chorion (*arrows*).

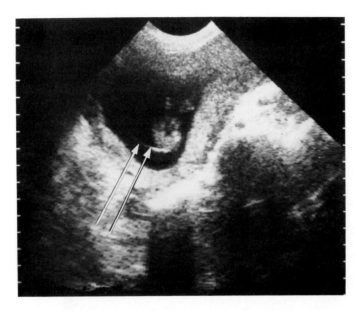

consists of a combination of the chorionic and amniotic cavities (primarily the former) and is surrounded by chorionic villi and decidual reaction.

The chorion soon divides into two portions, the chorion frondosum and the chorion laeve. The chorion frondosum forms the primordial placenta and is separated from the uterine wall by decidua basalis (Figure 3). The amniotic cavity enlarges and flattens out the chorionic cavity by about 10 weeks menstrual age (Figure 4). Between 7 and 10 weeks the yolk sac (Figure 5) can be identified in the chorionic cavity (9,15). Fusion of the amnion with the chorion is very often incomplete and one may see the amnionic membrane (Figure 6) as a distinct structure well into the second trimester. This may cause some diagnostic difficulty, particularly with subchorionic hemorrhage or twin abortion. When the amnion is not fused with the placenta, a sonolucent space is seen along the chorion plate. (These problems are also illustrated and discussed in Chapter 4, ''The Placenta.'')

At about 8 weeks after the last menstrual period, the disk-like shape of the gestation can be appreciated. The gestational sac usually has a thin wall facing the uterine cavity and a thick wall that includes chorion frondosum and decidua basalis attached to the uterus.

Figure 7

Blighted ovum. A gestational sac devoid of echoes.

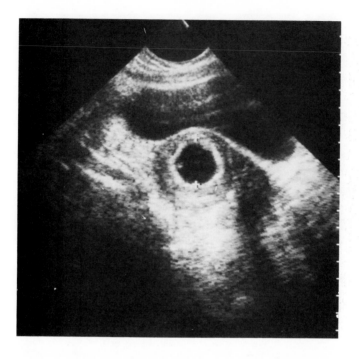

At 6 to 7 weeks, one should be able to see an embryo in the amniotic cavity, and with real-time equipment cardiovascular pulsation should be perceived. The gestational sac continues to grow and usually fills the entire uterine cavity at about the 11th week. The primordial placenta can frequently be identified as early as the 8th week but is relatively easy to see by the 11th or 12th week. By the 8th week, embryonic activity is consistently noted, and the fetal heart beat should always be seen using high speed real-time equipment. Beyond 12 weeks, no difficulty should be encountered in measuring the fetal head.

Threatened or missed abortion

Twenty percent of pregnant women bleed vaginally in the first trimester, but less than half of these are destined to abort. If abortion is preceded by sudden and profuse bleeding, often it must be dealt with under poorly controlled conditions. In order to avoid this potentially hazardous emergency situation, some investigators have attempted to use ultrasound to predict which jeopardized pregnancy will abort. Low lying, ill-defined, and double gestational sacs have been reported to correlate with an unfavorable

Figure 8

Arrow shows empty gestational sac of what is assumed to be a twin pregnancy. The other shows a live embryo.

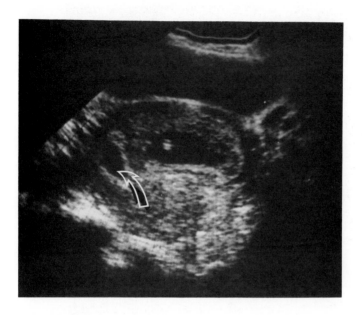

outcome. Others have associated ill-defined placentas and small-for-dates uteri and gestational sacs with abortion. In our experience none of these criteria consistently correlates with the outcome of pregnancy. Demonstration of an empty gestational sac after about 8 weeks is a reliable finding of a blighted ovum (Figure 7). Before one can conclude that the gestational sac contains no embryo, however, it must be thoroughly scanned with a high quality real-time device. Even when an embryo is present, it cannot be concluded that the gestation is viable unless cardiovascular pulsation is observed. The heart can be consistently seen at 7 weeks using a high resolution mechanical sector scanner with a frame rate of 20 Hz, as well as with new double-focused linear arrays, but each user must establish norms for the equipment he uses. As mentioned earlier an overfilled bladder may flatten the gestation sac and lead to an erroneous diagnosis of blighted ovum.

A common cause of first trimester bleeding is the blighted twin. In this situation one sac is empty and the other contains a viable embryo (Figure 8). In general the prognosis for the surviving embryo is excellent (3,13). The diagnosis can only be made with absolute certainty when two embryos have been observed and

Figure 9
Transonic area surrounded by echogenic rim.

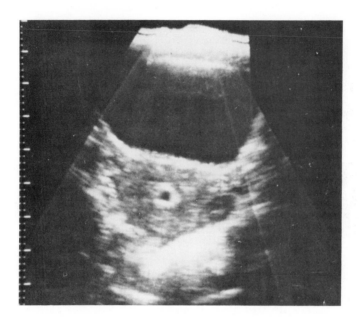

one dies or is expelled, so that its true incidence is unknown. When the first examination is carried out after one embryo has aborted, incomplete fusion of the amnion and chorion as well as subchorionic hemorrhage must be considered in the differential diagnosis.

When abortion has already occurred, multiple disorganized echoes are seen within the uterus. If abortion has been complete, the uterus may be indistinguishable from a non-pregnant uterus except for its size. Restoration of the cavity line suggests that curettage is probably not necessary, but we know of no data testing this hypothesis. The difference between incomplete abortion and missed abortion is perhaps more theological than practical, but in a missed abortion one is likely to see a gestation that is not in correspondence with the patient's dates and that shows no signs of life.

Ectopic pregnancy

Now that determinations of β subunits of hCG are available in most institutions, analysis of the problem of ectopic pregnancy can begin with confident knowledge of whether or not the patient is pregnant. If she is pregnant, the next question is, ''Is the pregnancy intrauterine or extrauterine?'' Unfortunately, the answer

Figure 10

a. Transverse scan demonstrating a transonic area within the uterus which is not surrounded by an echogenic rim (*straight arrow*). This patient had an ectopic pregnancy, and blood is visible in the cul-de-sac on the left side (*curved arrow*). *b.* Sagittal scan in the same patient showing blood in the cul-de-sac (*curved arrow*).

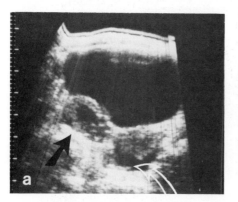 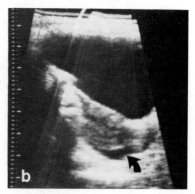

to that question is not always trivial. As suggested earlier, a gestation of 4 or 5 weeks may not yet be detectable and may well be accompanied by some adnexal abnormalities. On the other hand, in many patients with ectopic gestation there is a decidual cast or pseudogestational sac that can be difficult to distinguish from an intrauterine gestation (10). If there is an adnexal abnormality or fluid in the cul-de-sac, a pseudogestational sac must be strongly suspected.

Since the coexistence of intrauterine and ectopic pregnancies is a very rare event, the latter diagnosis can be effectively ruled out by conclusively demonstrating the former. Ultrasonic visualization of fetal cardiac activity within the uterus is undeniable evidence of an intrauterine pregnancy, but this can rarely be seen until 7 weeks' gestation or about 1 to 2 weeks after visualization of a gestational sac. Prior to the appearance of cardiac pulsation, the diagnosis hinges on the appropriateness of ultrasonic findings with respect to objective biochemical parameters. The urine pregnancy test is often misleading, and one cannot rely on the demonstration of an extrauterine mass in an early ectopic gestation. Moreover, many conditions such as pelvic inflammatory disease and ruptured ovarian cysts have sonographic findings similar to ectopic pregnancy.

Kadar et al. (8) have presented ultrasonic criteria for diagnosing healthy intrauterine pregnancies based on

Figure 11

Transverse scan showing a thickened but empty uterus (*straight arrow*). A gestational sac containing a live embryo was visible in the right tube (*curved arrow*).

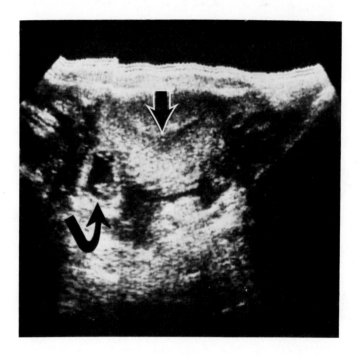

simultaneously determined serum hCG values. They define a normal gestational sac as a transonic area surrounded by an echogenic rim (Figure 9). In their series this ultrasonic finding in patients whose β subunit serum hCG values were in excess of 6000–6500 mIU/ml (the "discriminatory zone") was associated with normal intrauterine pregnancies. Either no intrauterine sac or a sac without an echogenic rim together with serum values above the discriminatory zone was found to be diagnostic of an ectopic pregnancy (Figure 10*a* and *b*).

The authors found that the sacs of intrauterine pregnancies usually did not become visible until the discriminatory zone was reached and, therefore, the absence of a sac with values below 6000 mIU/ml cannot distinguish between normal and abnormal gestations. When, however, a transonic area surrounded by an echogenic rim is present in association with serum hCG levels *below* 6000 mIU/ml, either a missed abortion or an ectopic pregnancy should be suspected, but a normal intrauterine pregnancy is very unlikely. An ectopic pregnancy in

Table 1
Possible Diagnoses Based on Serum Human Chorionic Gonadotropin (hCG) Levels and Sonar Findings from Patients with Suspected Ectopic Pregnancy*

Serum hCG Level (mIU/ml)	Ultrasound Findings	Diagnosis
Above discriminatory hCG zone†	Normal uterus / Decidual reaction / Transonic area	Ectopic pregnancy
	Intrauterine sac	Intrauterine pregnancy
Below discriminatory hCG zone‡	Normal uterus / Decidual reaction / Transonic area / Intrauterine sac	None
	Adnexal or cul-de-sac mass	Abnormal pregnancy§ / Ectopic pregnancy

* From Kadar, N., DeVore, G., and Romero, R.: Discriminatory hCG zone: Its use in the sonographic evaluation for ectopic pregnancy. Obstet. Gynecol. 58:2, 156, 1981.
† Greater than 6500 mIU/ml.
‡ Less than 6000 mIU/ml.
§ Missed abortion or ectopic pregnancy.

this setting becomes a more likely possibility if an adnexal mass can be visualized, but adnexal masses were found in only 42% of the ectopics in the series (Figure 11).

The findings in the study by Kadar et al. are summarized in Table 1. The group requiring follow-up studies when their scheme is used are those clinically stable patients whose scans show either an empty uterus or only a thin transonic sac in association with serum hCG levels less than 6000 mIU/ml. These women may have unruptured ectopic pregnancies or early normal pregnancies and should be followed with serial serum hCG determinations. In another study (7), Kadar and colleagues have shown that approximately 85% of patients with normal intrauterine pregnancies demonstrate an increase of 66% or more in serum hCG values obtained 48 hrs. apart, while those with ectopic pregnancies do not. By using the percentage increase over baseline values, the clinician is freed from trying to correlate serum hCG titers with a specific gestational age. This is useful because of the overlap of these values when normal and abnormal pregnancies are mixed. Furthermore, many women suspected of having ectopic pregnancies do not know the date of their last menstrual period.

While this scheme does not entirely eliminate laparoscopies for women who, in fact, have intrauterine

Figure 12

Transverse scan showing gestational sacs in both horns of a
bicornuate uterus.

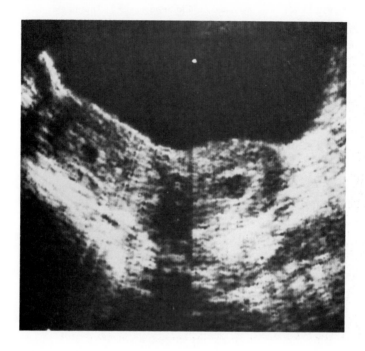

pregnancies or, alternatively, delays in the detection of
unruptured ectopics, we have found that it has
significantly decreased the incidence of both.

A false-positive diagnosis of ectopic pregnancy is
possible in some patients with bicornuate uteri since
the gestational sac is eccentrically placed (Figure 12).

Unusual locations of ectopic gestations must also be
considered. These include:
1   interstitial, characterized by an eccentrically placed
    gestation that does not have a complete myometrial
    mantle (6) (Figure 13).
2   cervical, fortunately exceedingly rare.
3   abdominal, usually a viable gestation that can be seen
    outside (1,5,17) the uterus. The uterus is compressed
    by the pregnancy, but the cavity line is visible. Although
    the absence of surrounding amniotic fluid often
    obscures the placental outline, the placenta may be
    remarkably well-defined. Other criteria listed by
    Allibone et al. (1) include absence of a uterine wall
    between the fetus or placenta and the bladder or the
    abdominal wall and localization of the placenta outside
    the uterine cavity (Figure 14).

Figure 13

Parasagittal scan of interstitial pregnancy. Note that the myometrial layer adjacent to the abdominal wall is virtually absent.

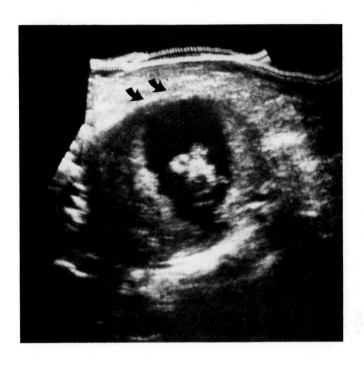

Hydatidiform mole

Hydatidiform mole is an important complication of early pregnancy, and ultrasound has become the definitive means of diagnosis. In roughly 50% of cases the uterus is larger than would be anticipated from menstrual history. The ultrasonic appearance of a mole reflects the gross pathological appearance. That is, the individual solid elements are separated by fluid spaces representing the myriad of vesicles of different size (Figure 15). Although the typical mole is easy to identify, about one-fourth of moles have an atypical appearance because they contain large blood clots or areas of cystic degeneration (4,14). Thus, they resemble incomplete abortions (Figure 16). With currently available ultrasonic equipment, there is no reliable way of distinguishing an atypical mole from an incomplete abortion, particularly at a very early stage, but a thick ring of echoes around the central sonolucent zone should suggest trophoblastic disease (19). The history, physical findings, and chorionic gonadotropin levels must be considered before one diagnoses a hydatidiform mole. Theca lutein cysts develop in response to the persistently high titers of chorionic gonadotropin in about one-half of cases, and

Figure 14

Sagittal scan showing a live intraabdominal pregnancy. Caudal to placenta is uterus. *a*, amniotic fluid; *curved arrow*, placenta; *straight arrow*, embryo.

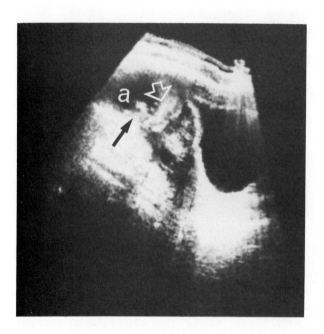

Figure 15

Typical mole with many vesicles of different size.

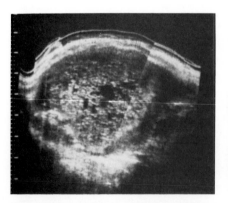
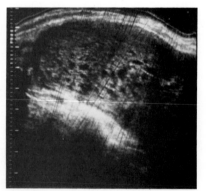

this finding may aid the ultrasonographer in the diagnosis of a mole.

Once the diagnosis is made by ultrasound it is imperative that the ultrasonographer's report be explicit

Figure 16

Early mole resembling incomplete abortion.

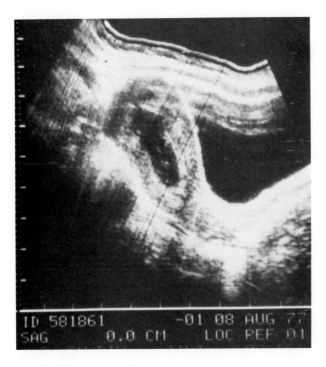

ID 581861   -01 08 AUG 77
SAG   0.0 CM   LOC REF 01

and leave no room for procrastination. It is not acceptable to suspect a diagnosis of a mole and request another ultrasound after an interval of time. Once it is established that the gestation is not viable, a curettage should be carried out.

Hydatidiform mole may coexist with pregnancy. In the so-called "incomplete" form there is a single placenta with functioning villous capillaries as well as hydatidiform swelling (Figure 17). The partial mole is often associated with a triploid fetus. A "complete" mole involves one of the placentas of a multiple gestation. In either case the molar tissue can be recognized as abnormal placenta. It is dense and homogenous with a few small liquid spaces corresponding to hydropic villi. The distinction is an important one because the incomplete mole is not considered a potentially malignant lesion (11,12,14,16,18).

The management of patients with a coexisting live fetus and mole is somewhat controversial. Most authorities suggest immediate evacuation, particularly since progressive symptoms of pre-eclampsia may begin in

Figure 17
Fetus with molar degeneration.

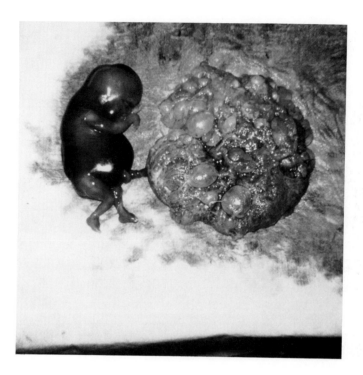

the second trimester. However, one author has carried a fetus to term in an asymptomatic mother since there is no evidence that this increases the risk of malignant degeneration (18). Some cases that resemble mole may be due to hydropic degeneration of the placenta, a condition of uncertain biological potential (11). In these cases hCG levels may be normal, and there are no accepted guidelines to clinical management.

In addition to the problem of mole masquerading as incomplete abortion, one is occasionally confronted with an incomplete abortion resembling a mole. Rarely, a degenerating uterine leiomyoma in a non-gravid woman may mimic a mole. In these patients there is a history of oligomenorrhea and the hCG titers are not elevated (12). There is no way to distinguish a choriocarcinoma from a benign mole with ultrasound.

Adnexal masses

A common problem in the first trimester of pregnancy is the association of ovarian and uterine masses. Ovarian cysts are frequently seen in the first trimester, and the patient is often referred with a suspected diagnosis of

Figure 18
Very large corpus luteum cyst.

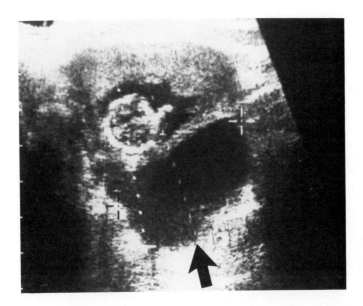

Figure 19
Multiple leiomyomata (*arrows*) displacing the placenta.

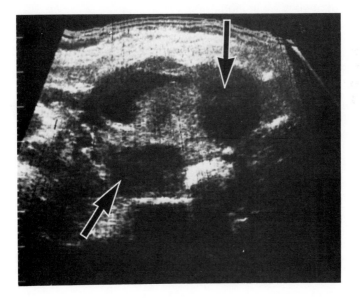

Figure 20

Midline sagittal section showing uterus with gestational sac. Superior to the uterus is a pelvic kidney.

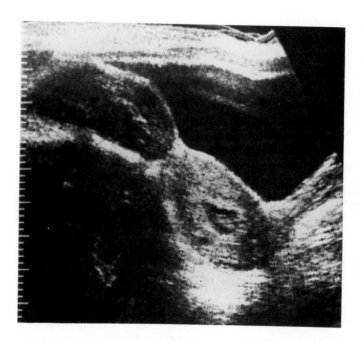

ectopic gestation. The patient and physician are both relieved of anxiety by demonstrating a normal intrauterine gestation associated with an ovarian cyst, thus excluding the diagnosis of an ectopic gestation. We have seen corpus luteum cysts (Figure 18) as large as 8 cm in diameter that disappeared during the second trimester. Uterine fibroids are also seen together with early pregnancies. Under these circumstances they are relatively echo-free and tend to displace the gestation from the anatomical center of the uterus. It is particularly characteristic to see the placenta displaced from the uterine wall by a fibroid (Figure 19).

Uterine leiomyomata may greatly increase in size during pregnancy and become edematous. Since edematous fibroids contain more water than adjacent tissue they are relatively non-attenuating, i.e., sonolucent. Rarely a fibroid undergoes such rapid growth during pregnancy as to undergo liquefactive necrosis, and such necrotic fibroids may resemble a mole. The leiomyoma must be distinguished from a transient uterine contraction (see Chapter 4, "The Placenta"). The latter does not have the typical whorled

Figure 21

Early intrauterine pregnancy in a patient wearing an IUD. Notice that the IUD extends into the cervical canal.

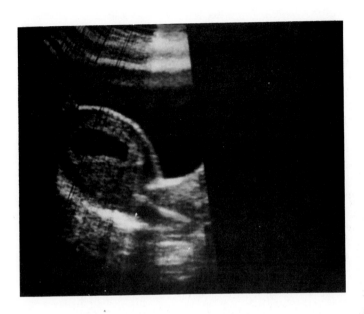

texture of the fibroid, and its superior and inferior borders are not well-defined.

A cystic teratoma or dermoid cyst is another tumor that may coexist with pregnancy. Its features are variable because of the wide variety of gross pathological appearance of this tumor, but it is often very echogenic because of hair, sebaceous material, and calcium. A pelvic kidney should not be mistaken for a pelvic tumor (Figure 20).

Pregnancy with intrauterine devices

An IUD is easily located by ultrasound in a non-pregnant uterus. Occasionally, a patient with an intrauterine device becomes pregnant, and the ultrasonographer is called upon to locate the IUD. In our experience in these cases it is extremely difficult to identify the IUD after the first trimester since the device attaches itself to the placenta or uterine wall. As the uterus grows, the IUD is drawn into the cavity and attains a lateral position between uterine wall and membranes (Figure 21) where it may be inaccessible to the ultrasound beam. Therefore, the inability to identify an intrauterine device in a pregnant patient does not exclude its presence nor does it indicate that it has perforated the uterine cavity. It is wise to perform an ultrasound examination as soon as possible in a patient with an IUD who suspects she is pregnant. Early removal of the IUD improves the prognosis of the pregnancy, which otherwise runs a high risk of septic abortion, and an unwanted pregnancy can be evacuated promptly.

References

1 **Allibone, B.W., Fagan, C.J., Porter, S.C.:** The sonographic features of intra-abdominal pregnancy. J. Clin. Ultrasound 9:383, 1981.

2 **Callen, P.W., DeMartini, W.J., Filly, R.A.:** The central uterine cavity echo: A useful anatomic sign in the ultrasonographic evaluation. Radiology 131:187, 1979.

3 **Finberg, H.J., Birnholz, J.C.:** Ultrasound observations in multiple gestation with first trimester bleeding: The blighted twin. Radiology 132:137, 1979.

4 **Fleischer, A.C., James, A.E., Jr., Krause, D.A., Millis, J.B.:** Sonographic patterns in trophoblastic diseases. Radiology 126:215, 1978.

5 **Graham, M.F.:** First trimester abdominal pregnancy. J. Clin. Ultrasound 5:321, 1977.

6 **Graham, M., Cooperberg, P.L.:** Ultrasound diagnosis of interstitial pregnancy: Findings and pitfalls. J. Clin. Ultrasound 7:433, 1979.

7 **Kadar, N., Caldwell, B.V., Romero, R.:** A method of screening for ectopic pregnancy and its indications. Obstet. Gynecol. 58:162, 1981.

8 **Kadar, N., DeVore, G., Romero, R.:** Discriminatory hCG zone: Its use in the sonographic evaluation for ectopic pregnancy. Obstet. Gynecol. 58:156, 1981.

9 **Mantoni, M., Pedersen, F.:** Ultrasound visualization of the human yolk sac. J. Clin. Ultrasound 7:459, 1979.

10 **Marks, W.M., Filly, R.A., Callen, P.W., Laing, F.C.:** The decidual cast of ectopic pregnancy: A confusing ultrasonographic appearance. Radiology 133:451, 1979.

11 **Munyer, T.P., Callen, P.W., Filly, R.A., Braga, C.A., Jones, H.W., III:** Further observations on the sonographic spectrum of gestational trophoblastic disease. J. Clin. Ultrasound 9:349, 1981.

12 **Naumoff, P., Szulman, A.E., Weinstein, B., Mazer, J., Surti, U.:** Ultrasonography of partial hydatidiform mole. Radiology 140:467, 1981.

13 **Robinson, H.P., Caines, J.S.:** Sonar evidence of early pregnancy failure in patients with twin conceptions. Br. J. Obstet. Gynaecol. 84:22, 1977.

14 **Santos-Ramos, R., Forney, J.P., Schwarz, B.E.:** Sonographic findings and clinical correlations in molar pregnancy. Obstet. Gynecol. 56:186, 1980.

15 **Sauerbrei, E., Cooperberg, P.L., Poland, B.J.:** Ultrasound demonstration of the normal fetal yolk sac. J. Clin. Ultrasound 8:217, 1980.

16 **Sauerbrei, E.E., Salem, S., Fayle, B.:** Coexistent hydatidiform mole and live fetus in the second trimester. Radiology 135:415, 1980.

17 **Sauerbrei, E., Toi, A., Effer, S.B., Fayle, B.W.K.:** Intrauterine to intraabdominal pregnancy: Ultrasound demonstration. Am. J. Roentgenol. Radium Ther. Nucl. Med. 133:132, 1979.

18 **Suzuki, M., Matsunobu, A., Wakita, K., Nishijima, M., Osanai, K.:** Hydatidiform mole with a surviving coexisting fetus. Obstet. Gynecol. 56:384, 1980.

19 **Woodward, R.M., Filly, R.A., Callen, P.W.:** First trimester molar pregnancy: Nonspecific ultrasonographic appearance. Obstet. Gynecol. 55:31S, 1980.

Estimation of Gestational Age

3

As might be surmised from the previous chapter on early gestation, gestational age between 6 and 12 weeks can be estimated from the size of the gestational sac. Robinson has made measurements of the volume of the gestational sac, but such measurements are beyond the constraints of time imposed in the average laboratory (11). Measurements of the uterus have also been made, but the variability of shape of the uterus in early pregnancy makes the selection of standard measurements difficult. Another method that has been used to estimate gestational age is crown-rump length (Figure 1). Robinson has shown that the length varies from 10 mm at 7 weeks to 85 mm at 14 weeks (see Appendix) (10). Because of the infinite variety of positions in which the very mobile fetus may lie in early gestations, the measurement of crown-rump length is difficult to make using contact equipment. Robinson employed multiple sections from which he selected the proper obliquity for measurement of the crown-rump length. His data show a fetal length-maturity curve which is quite impressive with an accuracy of plus or minus 3 days. Crown-rump length can be measured relatively easily when high resolution real-time equipment is used to locate the proper scanning plane and measurements are made from the frozen image with electronic calipers (Figure 2).* Inclusion of the yolk sac in the crown-rump length measurement will, of course, lead to an incorrect result. The crown-rump length and biparietal diameter are both available and useful between 11 and 13 weeks. Beyond 13 weeks the crown-rump length is much less reliable than the biparietal diameter.

The biparietal diameter (BPD) of the fetal skull is an excellent means of estimating gestational age in the second trimester because the measurement is subject to relatively little error, and there is a close correlation between biparietal diameter and gestational age. The

---

* A simple rule of thumb is that gestational age in weeks equals crown-rump length in centimeters + 6.

Figure 1

Use of electronic calipers to measure crown-rump length at 9.5 weeks.

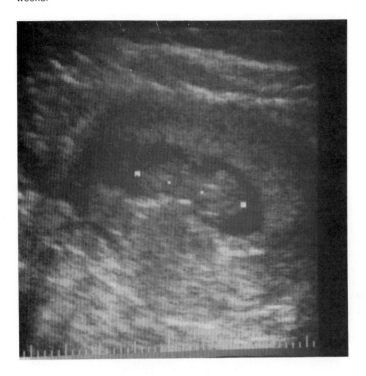

fetal skull is growing rapidly and is relatively thin. Thus, in the early second trimester a measurement error of 5 mm may correspond to only 1 week of growth, and the thinness of the fetal skull makes correction for velocity of sound in bone unnecessary. Another advantage of a thin fetal skull is that there is no ambiguity about the points from which measurements should be made. As the gestation progresses, the rate of fetal growth is reduced whereas the absolute accuracy of measurement is not improved. In addition, the correlation of biparietal diameter with gestational age is reduced as the pregnancy advances, i.e., the biological variability increases. Thus, the more advanced the pregnancy, the less reliable is the dating by biparietal diameter. In a patient in whom there is risk of growth retardation, measurement of the fetal head should begin at 16 to 20 weeks. Since the standard error of measurement of the biparietal diameter is about 2 mm and the growth of the biparietal diameter falls to about 1.5 mm/week in the last trimester, serial measurements of the biparietal diameter in the third trimester do not provide an adequate method of monitoring growth retardation. Moreover, as will be discussed in a subsequent chapter on fetal growth and development, retardation of fetal head growth occurs

Figure 2
BPD and crown-rump length of the same fetus at 12.5 weeks.

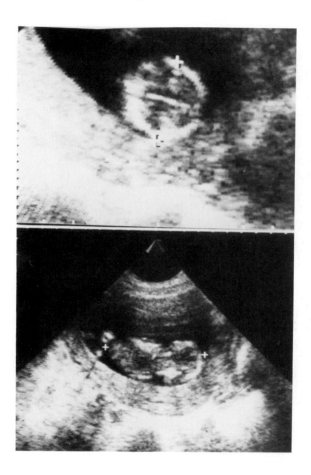

relatively late in the course of placental insufficiency.

Although the biparietal diameter is the mainstay for dating of the fetus, many limitations and problems must be considered.

1   Unrealistic accuracy of measurement should not be expected. A standard error of 2 mm is probably inherent in the selection and measurements of the BPD. A method that the individual user can employ to test his own reliability has been proposed by Davison et al. (1). That is, a series of measurements is made on the same patient 24 hrs. apart. They must, of course, be made without knowledge of the previous measurement. Since it can be assumed that no growth has occurred during the 24-hr. period, the standard deviation of the difference between the two measurements can be used as the "between occasion error."

Figure 3a

Axial section through "flattened" (dolichocephalic) head at the level of the thalami.

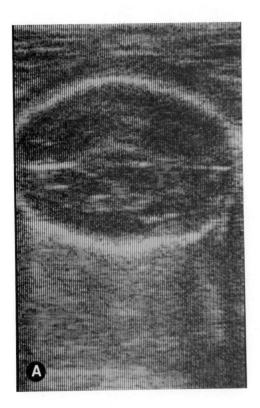

Figure 3b

Diagram of head showing the biparietal (*B.P.D.*) and occipito-frontal (*O.F.*) diameters.

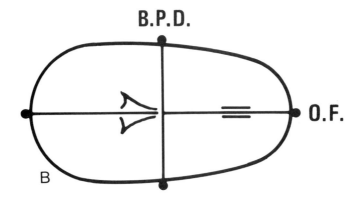

2   All of the existing charts of BPD were constructed before the anatomy of fetal brain displayed on sonograms was understood, and it is likely that the measurements were not all made from the same end points.

3   The fetal skull is compressible and occipitofrontal diameters (OFD) would be required to provide a more complete assessment of head size. Hadlock et al. (4) have shown that if the BPD/OFD is greater than 83% or less than 74%, the head is too wide or too long and the BPD is correspondingly misleading (Figure 3a and b). In such cases head circumference is a better index of gestational age. (Circumference is approximated by

$$\left(\frac{BPD + OFD}{2}\right) \times \pi)$$

4   There is biological variability in head growth. (Although altitude plays a role, race does not, at least in the North American population.) Sabbagha et al. have attempted to deal with the factor of biological variability by using the fetus as its own control (12). If two BPD measurements are made, the first at 18 to 26 weeks and the second at 30 to 33 weeks, the growth in the interval between the two measurements can be compared with the average growth. If growth has been significantly greater than average it is likely that the first BPD measurement was indeed made on a fetus whose head size was greater than average and thus younger (by 7 to 10 days) than the average gestational age corresponding to the initial BPD. Also, other things being equal, one would expect this fetus to continue to grow more rapidly than average and it can be placed on an above average expected growth curve. If, on the other hand, the growth between measurements has been less than average, the contrary argument can be made and the fetus was probably older (by 7 to 10 days) than the initial BPD suggested and can be placed on the below average growth curve. Fetuses in the latter group are more likely to be growth-retarded than the average and above average growers, whereas fetuses in the above average group are more likely to be macrosomic. More recently Tamura and Sabbagha (13) have divided abdominal growth similarly and by combining head and body growth characteristics divided fetuses into 3×3 or 9 groups (large, average, and small heads × large, average, and small bodies.)

The concept proposed by Sabbagha, growth-adjusted sonar age (GASA), thus has two functions. First, it refines the correlation of BPD with gestational age by a retrospective measurement of growth during a known time period. Second, it defines a subset of fetuses at risk for symmetrical growth retardation.

Although GASA provides added precision by dealing

with problem 4, it cannot eliminate problems 1, 2, and 3. Moreover, differences due to factors 1, 2, and 3 will affect GASA since it is no more accurate than the BPD measurements on which it is based.

GASA deals with gestational age, not date of delivery, but it is interesting that O'Brien et al. in a study of 50 patients who delivered spontaneously found no significant improvement in predicting estimated date of confinement (EDC) when two examinations at average times of 22 and 27 weeks were combined. The absolute error for a single measurement was 8.3 ± 7.1 days. With two measurements it was 8.4 ± 6.9 days (6).

The biparietal diameter is not the only index of fetal head size, but it is the easiest to measure and has been generally accepted. The occipital frontal diameter may also be measured, and formulae are available relating it to fetal weight and maturity (see Appendix). Garrett and Robinson use the cross-sectional area of the fetal skull as their index of the maturity after 28 weeks (see Appendix). This method, since it integrates a large number of diameters, is statistically superior to biparietal diameter measurement. (Area can be approximated by the formula $\pi \times$ BPD $\times$ OFD/4.) Some manufacturers now include in their machine devices for electronically computing area and perimeter. These facilitate the measurement of the fetal head, thorax, or abdomen.

Although there was some initial reluctance to use real-time scanning as the definitive means of measuring BPD, there can now be no doubt that it is superior to articulated scanning both because it permits the examiner to follow the fetal head or wait for it to turn in proper position and because an optimal cross section can much more easily be obtained thanks to the much higher sampling rate of real-time. Anyone who continues to use an articulated static scanner for BPD measurements is either a masochist or a hopeless reactionary. The BPD is by definition measured at the widest axial section of the skull. That level is probably located between the section that contains the cerebral peduncles and that which contains the bodies of the lateral ventricles. This intermediate section contains the rounded segments of the thalami between which may occasionally be seen the slit-like third ventricle (Figure 4). It also usually contains the cavum septi pellucidi which was formerly thought to be the third ventricle, and the Sylvian fissures. It is amusing to look back at

Figure 4

Axial section through the fetal head at the level of the thalami (*short arrows*) and third ventricle (*long arrow*). *Open arrows* show end points for measurement of the BPD.

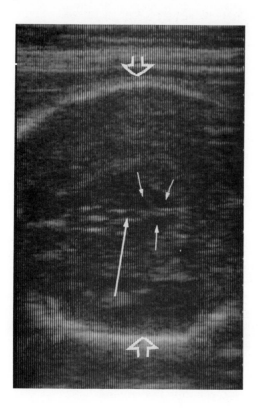

the first edition of this book in which we recommended the "third ventricle" as a landmark for the BPD. We were right for the wrong reasons. (This anatomy will be discussed in detail in Chapter 7 on fetal anatomy and congenital malformations.) We believe measurements made above and below that level tend to give slightly smaller values, although no systematic study of this problem has yet been published and this concept does not always accord with everyday experience.

Some positions of the fetal head simply do not permit a satisfactory biparietal diameter measurement. In such cases measurement of the intraorbital distance, which has shown an excellent correlation with gestational age, provides another cranial index (see Appendix) (Figure 5a and b). If the clinical situation is such that an approximate BPD is permissible, this should be obtained; but the report must stress that the measurement is only an approximation. Engagement of

Figure 5a

Axial section through the orbits in a fetus at 30 weeks. The lenses are seen anteriorly.

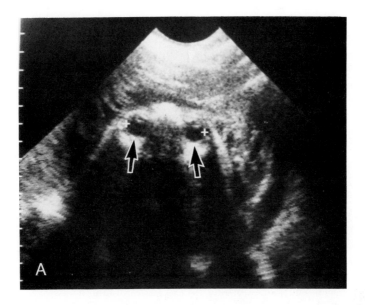

Figure 5b

Coronal section through the face of a fetus at 18 weeks showing orbits and facial bones.

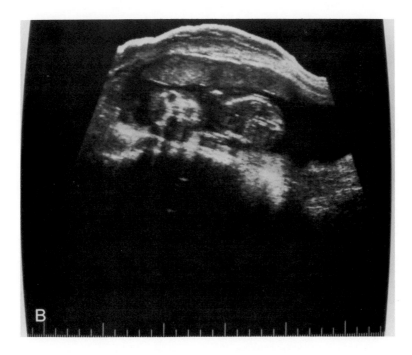

the fetal head also prevents adequate measurement of the biparietal diameter in some cases.

It should be pointed out that the methods used by different investigators to measure biparietal diameter are not identical. Most measurements of BPD are made from leading edge to leading edge. Anatomically, this means that one is measuring from the skin of the proximal side of the fetal head to the inner table of the distal side of the fetal skull. Some workers do not cut out the distal scalp; that is, they measure from the leading edge on the proximal side to the falling edge on the distal side. To add to the confusion, some who use leading edge measurements compensate for the scalp thickness as well as for the difference in velocity of sound in bone by calibrating their machines at 1600 meters/sec. rather than at 1540 meters/sec. (a difference of almost 4%, which results in the addition of about 3.5 mm in the full term fetal head). We feel that this "correction" compensates for two different problems in one imprecise way; that is, it makes all other measurements performed on the same machine 4% too large, and it ignores the fact that the thickness of the fetal skull is variable. For clinical purposes, however, absolute accuracy of measurement is not crucial as long as the method employed is consistent and the numbers have meaning in the laboratory in which they are used. In our Appendix we include tables of leading edge to leading edge and leading edge to falling edge.

In summary, the biparietal diameter, if carefully measured, is an accurate means of dating a pregnancy in the second trimester, but measurement of the BPD must not be elevated to a transcendental experience. For instance, a BPD within 10 days of the patient's dates is simply confirmatory evidence. To adjust the EDC by 10 days or less in such cases is ludicrous. If, however, dates and BPD are discordant by more than 1½ weeks, only three possibilities exist.

1 The measurement is wrong as a result of methodological problems.
2 The patient's dates are wrong. (This is very likely if there is a discrepancy of 4 weeks.)
3 Both the BPD and dates are correct, but head growth deviates significantly from normal.

One should try to dispel the ambiguity during the first examination rather than recommending serial scans in patients with questionable dates, since the latter policy is often wasteful and, at times, confusing.

1   Measurement error can occur when the BPD is calculated from a scan improperly obtained too high or low in the skull. This will result in an underestimation of gestational age. Underestimation can also result from cranial compression in multiple gestation, breech presentation, oligohydramnios, or a dolichocephalic skull with a BPD/OFD of less than 0.75.

Overestimation of fetal age can occur when one carelessly mistakes the occipito-frontal diameter for the BPD in a fetus presenting in an occiput anterior or posterior position. Attention to the intracranial and cranial anatomy should obviate this surprisingly frequent occurrence.

2   If careful review of a patient's scans fails to reveal a source of measurement error, the performance of additional fetal measurements should clarify the discrepancy between BPD and dates. Although AC or abdominal area calculations are not precise predictors of gestational age by themselves, they are very useful when combined with other data. For instance, if BPD suggests a fetal age of 32 weeks and the patient's dates are compatible with a 29-week gestation, an AC equal to a mean of 32 weeks would reinforce the operator's suspicion that the patient's dates were erroneous. If, additionally, a femur measurement accords with the other measurements, the case is clinched for mistaken dates. Obviously, it is possible that more information in some cases clouds, rather than clarifies, the picture when the measurements are discordant.

3   One should suspect an abnormality if dates and all other measurements are synchronous but the BPD is off by 3 weeks or more. For example, if the BPD is 3 weeks less than the AC, this body-to-head disproportion could be a result of microcephaly (especially if the patient's dates correlate with the AC). If, however, the BPD is 3 weeks or more ahead of the dates and other measurements, a thorough evaluation of intracranial anatomy should be undertaken since hydrocephaly could cause such a discrepancy.

Other abnormal conditions resulting in discrepancies in fetal measurements are asymmetrical intrauterine growth retardation in which BPD may be more than 3 weeks greater than AC or fetal macrosomia in which the AC is often 3 weeks ahead of BPD.

Measurement of femoral diaphyseal length is quite feasible with real-time instruments and has been

Figure 6

Both femurs in a fetus at 26 weeks. Notice that the anterior femur, but not the posterior, is seen in its entirety.

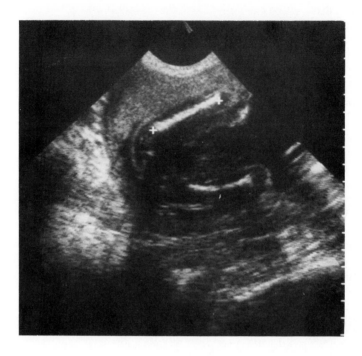

proposed as a method of dating the fetus (Figure 6) (2, 3, 5, 7–9) (see Appendix). Although femoral length correlates well with BPD, its measurement relies on the lateral rather than the axial resolution of the ultrasonoscope and is thus inherently less accurate. In addition, the difficulty of identifying the "true" length of the femur is greater than that of measuring the "true" BPD. The latter has definite anatomical landmarks, whereas the former depends on obtaining the largest measurement that can be consistently made. As will be discussed in the section on fetal anatomy and malformations, the measurement of femoral length is of use in the diagnosis of various types of skeletal malformations. However, if microcephaly or other cranial anomaly is suspected or the head is unmeasurable, the length of the femur can serve as the "gold standard."

References

1   **Davison, J.M., Lind, T., Farr, V., Whittingham, J.A.**: The limitations of ultrasonic fetal cephalometry. J. Obstet. Gynaecol. Br. Commonw. 80:769, 1973.

2   **Farrant, P., Meire, H.B.**: Ultrasound measurement of fetal limb lengths. Br. J. Radiol. 54:660, 1981.

3   **Filly, R.A., Golbus, M.S., Carey, J.C., Hall, J.G.**: Short-limbed dwarfism: Ultrasonographic diagnosis by mensuration of fetal femoral length. Radiology 138:653, 1981.

4   **Hadlock, F.P., Deter, R.L., Carpenter, R.J., Park, S.K.**: Estimating fetal age: Effect of head shape on BPD. Am. J. Roentgenol. 137:83, 1981.

5   **Hohler, C.W., Quetel, T.A.**: Comparison of ultrasound femur length and biparietal diameter in late pregnancy. Am. J. Obstet. Gynecol. 141:759, 1981.

6   **O'Brien, W.F., Coddington, C.C., Cefalo, R.C.**: Serial ultrasonographic biparietal diameters for prediction of estimated date of confinement. Am. J. Obstet. Gynecol. 138:467, 1980.

7   **O'Brien, G.D., Queenan, J.T.**: Growth of the ultrasound fetal femur length during normal pregnancy. Am. J. Obstet. Gynecol. 141:833, 1981.

8   **O'Brien, G.D., Queenan, J.T., Campbell, S.**: Assessment of gestational age in the second trimester by real-time ultrasound measurement of the femur length. Am. J. Obstet. Gynecol. 139:540, 1981.

9   **Queenan, J.T., O'Brien, G.D., Campbell, S.**: Ultrasound measurement of fetal limb bones. Am. J. Obstet. Gynecol. 138:297, 1980.

10 **Robinson, H.P.**: Sonar measurement of fetal crown-rump length as a means of assessing maturity in first trimester pregnancy. Br. Med. J. 4:28, 1973.

11 **Robinson, H.P.**: "Gestation sac" volumes as determined by sonar in the first trimester of pregnancy. Br. J. Obstet. Gynaecol. 82:100, 1975.

12 **Sabbagha, R.E., Hughey, M., Depp, R.**: Growth adjusted sonographic age (GASA): A simplified method. Obstet. Gynecol. 51:383, 1978.

13 **Tamura, R.K., Sabbagha, R.E.**: Percentile ranks of sonar fetal abdominal circumference measurements. Am. J. Obstet. Gynecol. 138:475, 1980.

The Placenta   **4**

The placenta is readily imaged with ultrasound, but
some problems in interpretation of the images are
worthy of detailed discussion. These include
localization of the placenta, confusing appearances,
"lesions" and normal variants, placenta previa,
abruption of the placenta, placental maturation and its
morphological features, and placental changes in
hydrops, diabetes, hypertension, and intrauterine
growth retardation (IUGR).

Operational localization of the placenta is desirable if
one wishes to avoid traversing it with a needle or
scalpel, or to obtain a fetal blood sample from the
placenta, and in the diagnosis of placenta previa.
However, classification of the placenta as anterior,
posterior, fundal, low, etc. is a useless exercise in
medical compulsiveness and is both imprecise and
misleading except insofar as it refers to the location at
the time of the scan and with the degree of distention of
the urinary bladder that was obtained when the scan
was made. Rotation of the uterus by the bladder and
asymmetrical uterine growth both alter placental
position, often unpredictably.

Placental appearance

The identification of the placenta with modern gray
scale (either dynamic or static) instruments is rarely a
problem unless there is very severe oligohydramnios.
The fetal surface is bordered by a strong specular
reflection referred to as the "chorionic plate." * In fact,
this reflection is produced by the amnionic membrane
covering the chorionic plate of the placenta, and in the
early second trimester fusion between the amnion and
chorion is often incomplete so that the ultrasonic
"chorionic plate" appears to be floating loosely in the
amniotic fluid (Figure 1). Between the amnion and
chorion there are many large fetal vessels that
anastomose with the umbilical vein at the locus of
attachment of the cord. These veins are often called
placental cysts, but if one observes them carefully with
high quality real-time equipment, blood flow can be
observed in the direction of the cord and the network of

---

* This is a misnomer "up with which we shall have to put," as Winston
Churchill would have said.

Figure 1

Second trimester anterior placenta showing incomplete fusion of amnion and chorion.

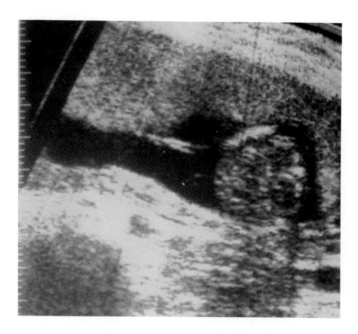

vessels can be followed deep into the substance of the placenta (9) (Figure 2). Occasionally, there is mucoid material in this region that is echo-free but does not exhibit blood flow.

The basal or maternal aspect of the placenta rests on the decidua basilis and a lacy appearing network of uterine veins (3, 8) (Figure 3). These vessels are best seen when the placenta is posterior and as it curves up from the posterior wall of the uterus to the fundus. They are not seen anterior to an anteriorly placed placenta unless a water path system is used because of reverberations from the skin and the poor resolution close to the transducer surface. The network of decidual and uterine veins also shows blood flow with real-time viewing and occasionally is a landmark to distinguish placenta from a region of transient uterine contractions that may resemble the placenta.

Within the placenta are sonolucent spaces of variable size that show a flow pattern. The larger spaces have a unique flow pattern characterized by arterial jets at the maternal rate and a whirlpool motion terminating in accelerating flow at the opposite pole of the space. This flow pattern indicates that the larger spaces are, in fact, venous lakes fed by uterine arteries and drained by placental veins (Figure 4).

Figure 2

Entrance of umbilical vein into the placenta with prominent veins shown (*arrow*).

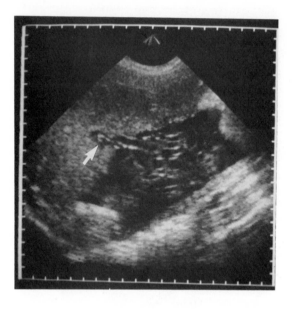

Figure 3

Decidual and uterine veins behind a posterior placenta (*arrows*).

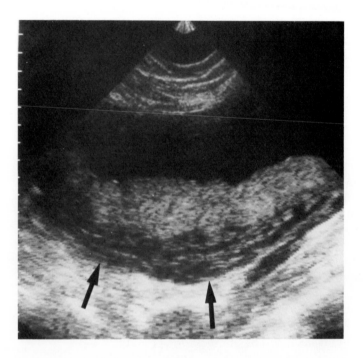

Figure 4
Venous lakes in placenta.

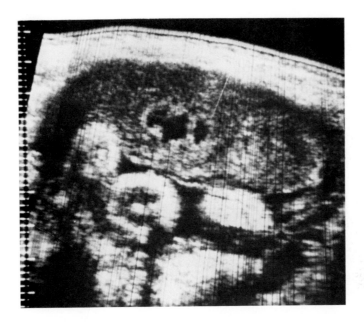

The various vascular spaces—including the veins
between the amnion and chorion, the basal veins, and
intraplacental venous lakes—are all normal structures.
Even large venous lakes have no clinical consequences
(Figure 5) that we know of, and the basal reticulum of
vessels should not be misinterpreted as evidence of
placental abruption (Figure 3).

Placental localization

Since the placenta is easy to localize, it would seem
that the diagnosis of placenta previa by ultrasound
should be trivial (Figures 6 and 7). Unfortunately this is
not the case for three reasons:

1   The location of the cervix is not always precisely
known, and an overfilled bladder may elongate the
lower end of the uterus so much that the internal os
appears to be much higher than it really is. It has been
suggested that the cervix should never be longer than
6 cm., and this measurement has been used by Zemlyn
as a successful guideline for the highest possible
position of the internal os (15). Another approach is to
repeat the scan after emptying of the bladder. This
maneuver reduces the pressure on the lower uterine
segment and may even result in rotation of the uterus
and placenta round its long axis.

Figure 5
Large venous lakes in a pregnancy with an uneventful outcome.

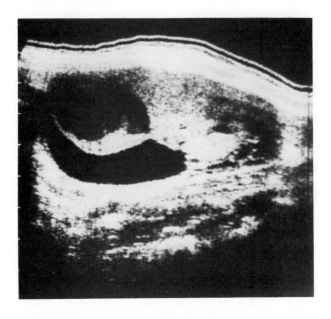

Figure 6
Anterior placenta previa.

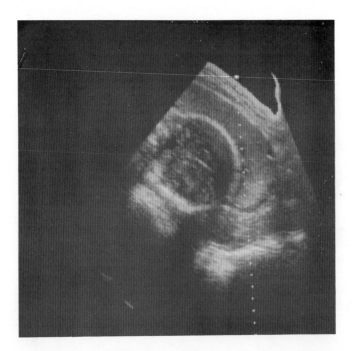

Figure 7
Posterior placenta previa.

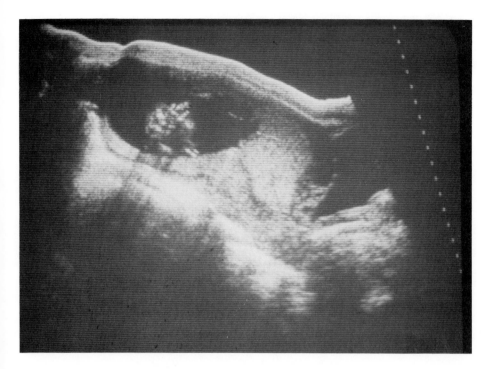

2   When the placenta is posterior and the fetus is in
    cephalic presentation, the fetal head shadows the
    posterior placenta so that its inferior extent cannot be
    seen. In this situation the head should be lifted out of
    the pelvis manually or the patient put in Trendelenberg
    position so as to provide an acoustic window into the
    cervix (2). Whether this space contains amniotic fluid or
    placenta will then be evident. Some placentas are
    primarily posterolateral, and their relation to the cervix
    is not visible in an anterior midline sagittal scan (6).
    They can only be imaged with oblique scans, a
    maneuver that is not difficult with real-time instruments
    (Figure 8).
3   The relationship of the placenta to the cervix changes
    as the pregnancy progresses (Figure 9). Fortunately,
    this change is always up toward the fundus, not down
    to the cervix. We have *never* seen a second trimester
    fundal placenta become previa at term. However, a
    very large number of apparently low second trimester
    placentas become fundal placentas by term. Wexler
    and Gottesfeld found that it was possible to exclude
    cases of second trimester "previa" from consideration
    if the "previa" was incomplete (i.e., did not encircle the
    cervix) or relinquished its position after emptying of the
    bladder (13). In the remainder of the cases—those that

Figure 8

Oblique scan showing a posterior placenta previa shielded by fetal head. A small portion of placenta is seen covering the internal os. This scan was made possible by angling the transducer.

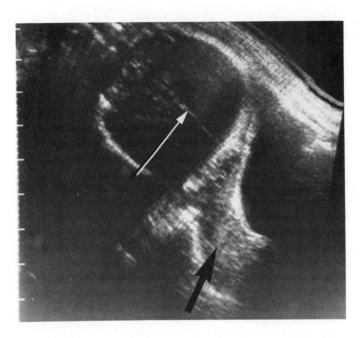

Figure 9

Second trimester "placenta previa." In subsequent scans the placental position with respect to the cervix changed, and the patient delivered vaginally at term.

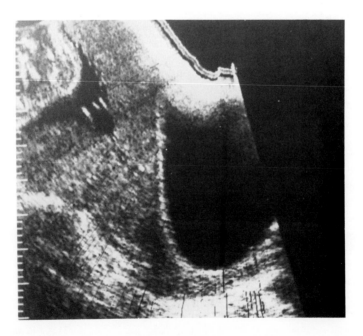

were complete and unrelenting, comprising 5.6% of the initial study group of 859 patients—the incidence of clinical previa at term was 12.5%. Ballas et al. (1) have shown that second trimester previa is more likely to result in clinical previa when accompanied by bleeding than when asymptomatic. Thirteen of 17 of their symptomatic second trimester cases of previa were terminated by cesarean section due to bleeding.

In order not to cause either undue anxiety or mismanagement of the patient, the ultrasonographer should follow these guidelines:

1. Second trimester asymptomatic partial "previa" can be ignored. It is not necessary to suggest multiple repeat examinations in these women.
2. If the previa appears complete either with an empty bladder or with the cervix considered to be no more than 6 cm. long, follow-up should be done before delivery. Under no circumstances should a decision about management be based on an examination that is more than 2 weeks old.
3. Symptomatic second trimester previas should be followed until the placental position changes or the patient delivers. Their clinical management should also be expectant.
4. Term or near-term patients with low lying posterior or posterolateral placentas must be scanned by some method that allows one to visualize both the cervix and placenta. This may include oblique or lateral scans and elevation of the fetal head. The linear array is not the best instrument in these doubtful cases. One should not be reassured by the fact that most of the placenta is in the fundus. The placenta may be long or bilobed (Figure 10). If there is persistent doubt, a "double set-up" is indicated.

Placental abruption

The diagnosis of placental abruption can often be made when blood dissects retroplacentally without forming a hematoma and elevates the chorioamniotic membrane (12) (Figure 11). In the early second trimester this appearance is difficult to distinguish from incomplete fusion of the amnion and chorion. However, we have seen women with bleeding who had this finding and in whom genetic amniocentesis done some weeks later showed old blood in the amniotic fluid. Fortunately, elevation of the membranes is not necessarily a sign of a large abruption and pregnancies with this finding generally progress uneventfully. Our experience with large retroplacental hematomas is very limited (Figure 12). Clotted blood adjacent to the placenta (Figure 13) may be seen with retroplacental or marginal sinus bleeding and may cover the cervix, simulating a placenta previa.

Figure 10
Bilobed placenta, the lower portion of which is a complete previa.

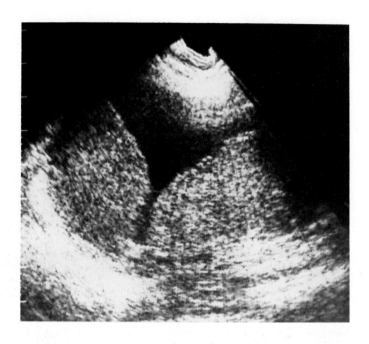

Figure 11
Retroplacental clot (*curved arrow*) elevating the membranes (*arrow*). This was observed in a patient at 18 weeks who presented with bleeding. This pregnancy proceeded uneventfully to term.

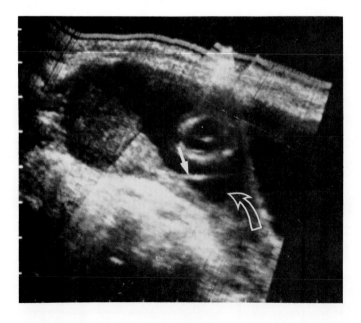

Figure 12

A large retroplacental clot in a patient at 22 weeks (*arrow*).

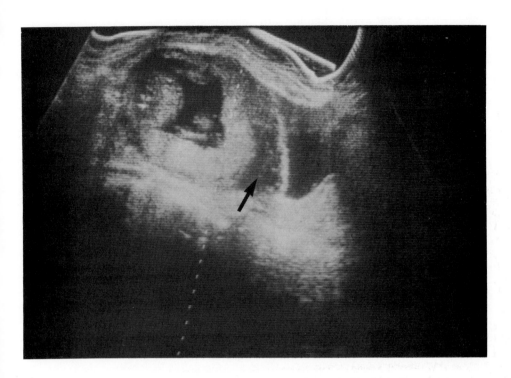

Figure 13

Clotted blood adjacent to anterior placenta mimicking a placenta previa.

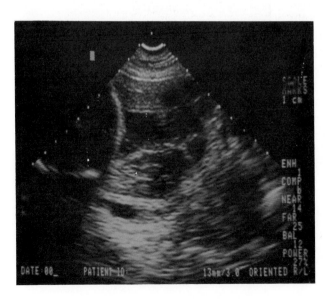

Placental infarcts are similar in their appearance to infarcts of other parenchymal organs. During the hemorrhagic phase they are relatively sonolucent but later undergo organization and calcification, thus resembling the changes in the mature placenta described below.

Placental morphology

One of the most interesting aspects of ultrasound placentography has been the study of placental maturity and senility, because these changes reflect the placenta's supply line and seem to be related to conditions not primary to the placenta itself.

In 1928 Schonig first described the presence of calcium in the placenta (11). If the calcium contained within granules was microscopic he called it "physiologic calcification." Gross calcification was considered "dystrophic calcification." Masters and Clayton in 1940 (7) performed in vivo placental x-ray studies and also attempted with clinical analysis to quantify placental calcium content. Their simplified classification of calcium deposition consisted of "none, some, much, and very much." It is of note that rarely was "very much" calcium found before 38 weeks and that the amount of calcification did not seem to correlate with the presence or absence of the postmaturity syndrome. Calcium deposition, however, did seem to occur in regions of villous degeneration close to the maternal placental surface.

Russell and Fielden (1969) found that only 19% of patients studied had radiological evidence of placental calcification in utero compared with 75 to 90% of placentas studied after birth (10).

Winsberg (1973) using ultrasound observed that placentas were either homogeneous or "irregular" in texture and the latter type of placenta was rarely noted before the 35th week of gestation. He noted echo-free "holes" in the placenta that seemed to conform in vitro to blood-filled central positions of the fetal cotyledon (14). Fisher et al. also described a "reticular" pattern of echoes that might or might not occur after 36 weeks of gestation (4). If seen before 36 weeks, this reticular texture often was noted in association with IUGR.

In 1979 Grannum et al. reported on a system of placental classification based on changes demonstrable by ultrasound (5) (Figures 14 and 15). According to this system, placentas can be graded according to the appearance of echo patterns in three areas: the basal zone, the chorionic plate, and the

Figure 14

Diagram showing the ultrasonic appearance of a grade 0, grade I, grade II, and grade III placenta.

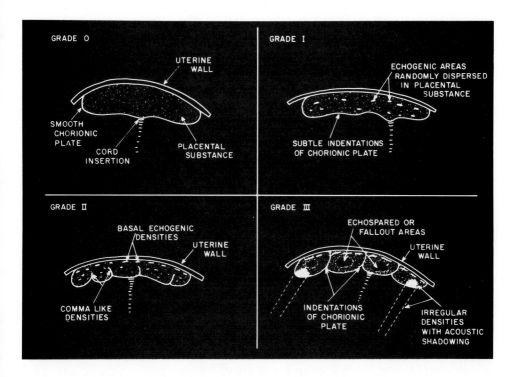

intervening placental substance (9). Grade 0 placentas are seen before the 28th week of gestation and rarely thereafter. The placenta is very homogeneous with a conspicuous absence of high level echoes anywhere in the placental substance. The chorionic plate in an anterior placenta is a straight line. In a grade 1 placenta echoes may be seen within the placental substance, and the chorionic plate attains an undulating appearance. The basal plate is not sharply outlined. Grade 1 placentas may be observed at any time in gestation. In one study, grade 1 placentas comprised approximately 40% of cases at term (5). A grade 2 placenta is distinguished by the presence of linear echoes that run parallel to the basal plate. The stippled echoes within the placental substance are often confluent, resulting in thick speckling. The chorionic plate may or may not have indentations. Approximately 40% of term placentas were of grade 2 morphology in the above-mentioned study.

The grade 3 placenta is the easiest to identify because of its characteristic compartmentalized appearance. Individual placental cotyledons are outlined by calcified

Figure 15

Composite of scans representing the four grades (note that these were taken from different patients).

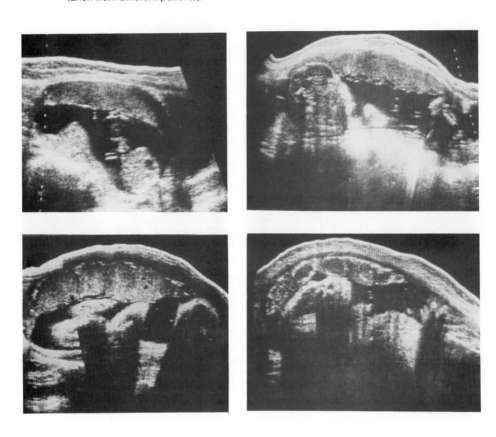

intercotyledonary septa. At least two cotyledons must be identified before the placenta is classified as grade 3. Sonolucent regions are often noted in the center of the isolated compartments, but this is not an invariable finding.

Grade 3 placentas were found in 15 to 20% of term patients in the study by Grannum et al. (5), and in our collective experience are rarely noted before the 36th week of gestation. Exceptions to this observation include patients with hypertension or those whose fetuses have intrauterine growth retardation. These patients comprise about 50% of those with "premature placental senescence," and the remaining 50% are patients wih completely normal pregnancies. If we identify a grade 3 placenta before 36 weeks, fetal and maternal surveillance is begun through non-stress testing and careful monitoring of maternal blood pressure. Often, this unusual ultrasound finding precedes the clinical emergence of hypertension by a week or more.

Although placental grading is greatly facilitated when the placenta is anterior, it is still possible to grade most fundal and posterior placentas. However, the combination of oligohydramnios and a posterior placenta precludes evaluation of placental morphology since the crowded fetus will completely shadow the underlying placenta.

The technique suggested when evaluating a posterior placenta is to scan sagitally over the area of the fetal extremities. Segments of the placenta can be seen between the limbs. Also, an angulated scan through a lateral window opposite the fetal body will permit access to portions of the posterior placenta.

Grannum et al. have correlated placental grading with pulmonic maturity (5). In their study L/S ratios were obtained in patients whose placentas were graded at the time of amniocentesis. L/S ratios were greater than 2.0 in 100% of patients with grade 3 placentas, 87% of patients with grade 2 placentas, and 68% of cases when a grade 1 placenta was found.

Since publishing the above study in 1979 we have been clinically correlating the finding of grade 3 placentas with neonatal outcomes in patients attending the comprehensive maternal care program at Yale-New Haven Hospital. As yet no infant has developed respiratory distress syndrome after a grade 3 placenta was shown by ultrasound. This association has held for infants born as early as 30 weeks of gestation. Although it would be unlikely that any diagnostic test will prove to have a 100% correlation with pulmonic maturity, we strongly suspect from this experience (and that of others) that placental grading will add an important guideline to the assessment of fetal pulmonic maturity.

About 7% of patients are undelivered by the 42nd week of gestation. These post-term gravidas have a 15% chance of harboring a fetus with postmaturity syndrome, a diagnosis based on the presence of meconium-stained amniotic fluid and decreased subcutaneous fat (resulting in wrinkled skin). Other more variable signs include long finger nails, lanugo, and decreased vernix. Perhaps the most consistent findings in postmaturity syndrome include morbidity from meconium aspiration, perinatal asphyxia, and thermal instability. Some studies suggest that postmature babies have an increased rate of adverse neurological sequelae.

Since it has been suggested that postmaturity syndrome is a phenomenon resulting from the inability of an aging placenta to support a demanding fetus, preliminary ultrasound studies of placental morphology in post-term patients are yielding some interesting information. In an ongoing study at Yale-New Haven Hospital, about 85% of pregnancies complicated by the post-maturity syndrome have grade 3 placentas. In the remaining 15%, grade 2 placentas were present. Not only were grade 1 placentas not associated with postmaturity syndrome, but they were not seen in any pregnancy documented to be more than 42 weeks. This interesting preliminary finding has been useful in identifying those patients thought to be at 42 weeks whose dates are in error.

Placentas in patients with fetal hydrops and diabetes have characteristic abnormalities discussed in Chapter 5, "Third Trimester Complications."

Accurate identification of textural and dynamic changes in the placenta requires equipment of high resolution and wide dynamic range. In the past such equipment has been necessarily static, but real-time units with these features are now generally available although not yet widely used. It should also be kept in mind that the linear array is not as good at providing access to posterior and fundal segments of the placenta as a mechanical sector scanner or articulated static scanner. Development of better ultrasonic instruments and measurement of other acoustic parameters than amplitude may also provide fascinating information about the placenta. Doppler, which has been used to measure umbilical vein flow, may also be valuable in studying intraplacental flow.

References

1 **Ballas, S., Gitstein, S., Jaffa, A.J., Peyser, M.R.**: Midtrimester placenta previa: Normal or pathologic finding. Obstet. Gynecol. 54:12, 1979.

2 **Bernstine, R.L., Lee, S.H., Crawford, W.L., Shimek, M.P.**: Sonographic evaluation of the incompetent cervix. J. Clin. Ultrasound 9:417, 1981.

3 **Callen, P.W., Filly, R.A.**: The placental-subplacental complex: A specific indicator of placental position on ultrasound. J. Clin. Ultrasound 8:21, 1980.

4 **Fisher, C.C., Garrett, W., Kosoff, G.**: Placental aging monitored by gray scale echography. Am. J. Obstet. Gynecol. 124:483, 1976.

5 **Grannum, P.A.T., Berkowitz, R.L., Hobbins, J.C.**: The ultrasonic changes in the maturing placenta and their relation to fetal pulmonic maturity. Am. J. Obstet. Gynecol. 133:915, 1979.

6 **Laing, F.C.**: Placenta previa: Avoiding false-negative diagnoses. J. Clin. Ultrasound 9:109, 1981.

7   **Masters, M., Clayton, S.C.**: Calcification of the human placenta. J. Obstet. Gynaecol. Br. Emp. 47:437, 1940.

8   **McGahan, J.P., Phillips, H.E., Reid, M. H.**: The anechoic retroplacental area. Radiology 134:475, 1980.

9   **Morin, F., Winsberg, F.**: Real-time identification of blood flow in the placenta and umbilical cord. J. Clin. Ultrasound. 10:1, 21, 1982.

10 **Russell, J.G.B., Fielden, P.**: The antenatal diagnosis of placental calcification. J. Obstet. Gynaecol. Br. Commonw. 76:813, 1969.

11 **Schonig, A.**: Über den Kalktransport von Mutter und Kind und über Kalkablagerung in der Plazenta. Z. Geburtshilfe Gynäkol. 94:451, 1928.

12 **Spirt, B.A., Kagan, E.H., Rozanski, R.M.**: Abruptio placenta: Sonographic and pathologic correlation. Am. J. Roentgenol. Radium Ther. Nucl. Med. 133:877, 1979.

13 **Wexler, P., Gottesfeld, K.R.**: Early diagnosis of placenta previa. Obstet. Gynecol. 54:231, 1979.

14 **Winsberg, F.**: Echographic changes with placental aging. J. Clin. Ultrasound 1:52, 1973.

15 **Zemlyn, S.**: The length of the uterine cervix and its significance. J. Clin. Ultrasound 9:267, 1981.

Third Trimester Complications

5

Introduction

Perinatal mortality rates have dropped appreciably over the past 10 years, largely through improved diagnostic methods. Occasionally, ultrasound allows the obstetrician to make decisions that may be urgently required in the third trimester patient, and the portability of smaller real-time machines makes them ideal for bedside examinations. This chapter deals with ultrasound's role in the management of a variety of pregnancy complications.

Abnormal fetal presentation

In obese or uncooperative patients, the classical Leopold abdominal maneuvers may be inadequate to diagnose fetal presentation. Even a pelvic examination may not reveal which fetal pole is in the pelvis. In such instances, a real-time examination provides the physician with exact knowledge of the fetal presentation. In a transverse lie, one can tell whether the back is up or down, and by scanning the lower uterus one can locate a previously undiagnosed placenta previa. Since cesarean section is the method of delivery for a viable fetus in a transverse lie, information about the position of the limbs and placenta is extremely useful to the physician about to enter the uterus through the lower uterine segment. In fact, to eliminate surprises, we routinely scan all intrapartum patients just prior to performing cesarean sections.

It is becoming common practice to deliver patients by cesarean section who present with a breech between 26 and 36 weeks (Figures 1 and 2) in order to minimize the morbidity associated with a vaginal delivery. The probable reason for the high rate of trauma associated with vaginal delivery in very low birth weight infants is that prior to 32 to 34 weeks the head circumference is larger than the lower body circumference (as indicated by head-to-body ratios) (5). Since the cervix is often incompletely dilated during delivery of the body of a small premature breech, the head, being larger by comparison, may become hung up during its passage through the cervix. Therefore, validation of gestational

Figure 1

Sagittal scan of a fetus in breech presentation at 30 weeks.

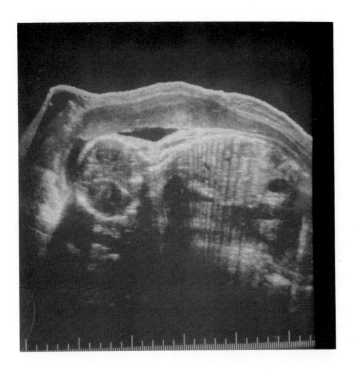

age with ultrasound is critical to the patient's management. Also, estimation of fetal weight is important when deciding the route of delivery for the patient with a breech. If, for example, estimated fetal weight is greater than 3500 g, we would strongly suggest delivery by cesarean section (13).

The BPD of a breech may be somewhat compressed (Figure 3 in Chapter 3) causing the unwary observer to conclude that the fetus is younger than its true age. Also, since the BPD is an important variable in the determination of fetal weight, the above phenomenon can result in underestimation of fetal weight. The additional measurement of occipital-frontal diameter (OFD) should help avoid underestimating fetal age and weight. If BPD is more than 75% of the OFD, the BPD is not significantly misleading. In dolichocephaly, however, the BPD is less than 75% of the OFD and underestimates gestational age (12). Head

Figure 2

Sagittal scan of a footling breech near term. Notice the umbilical cord (*C*) in the lower uterine segment and the potential for prolapse. *B*, bladder, *F*, foot.

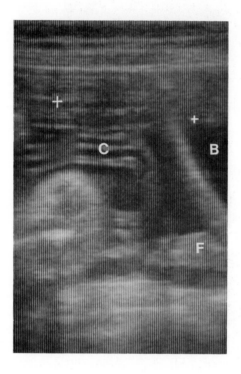

circumference measurements can also be used in these circumstances $HC = \dfrac{BPD + OFD}{2} \times \pi$.

In the large breech the use of ultrasound can avert later infant morbidity resulting from trauma to the aftercoming head due to cephalopelvic disproportion. Therefore, an estimation of the size of the fetal head and maternal pelvis is essential. At Yale, if the BPD is more than 9.6 cm, we deliver all patients by cesarean section irrespective of the size of the maternal pelvis. If the BPD is of moderate size (9.0 to 9.6 cm), the pelvis is measured by x-ray pelvimetry, and if any of the measurements are not adequate, cesarean section is performed.

Occasionally, an extended head is identified by x-ray pelvimetry. This finding alone is an indication for cesarean section since transection of the spinal cord can result from vaginal delivery when the fetal head is

Figure 3a

Sagittal scan of a face presentation. Notice the distortion of the cranial outline.

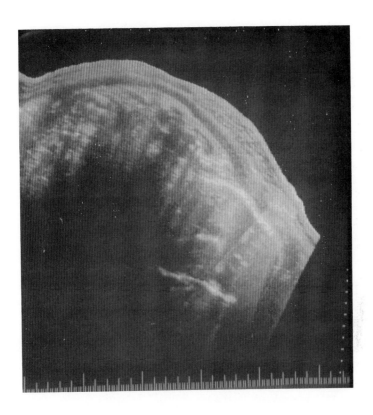

extended. Unlike the flexed fetus in a vertex presentation, the fetal head in a breech presentation will often be at about a 90° angle with the body (military position). Abnormal extension occurs when the head-to-body angle is more than 90°. With ultrasound this angle can be determined by scanning across the body until most of the abdominal aorta can be seen in one plane. This plane represents the long axis of the body. The end of the transducer on the occiput should be fixed and the other end rotated until the head appears as an elongated ellipse. This plane represents the long axis of the fetal head. The angle between these two axes approximates the angle of inclination of the head. This type of evaluation is possible only when the fetus is on its side. If an extended head is suspected by this ultrasound, it should be confirmed with a radiograph.

Fortunately, face presentations are rarely encountered. The diagnosis is usually made by pelvic examinations

Figure 3b

Transverse scan of the skull of this fetus.

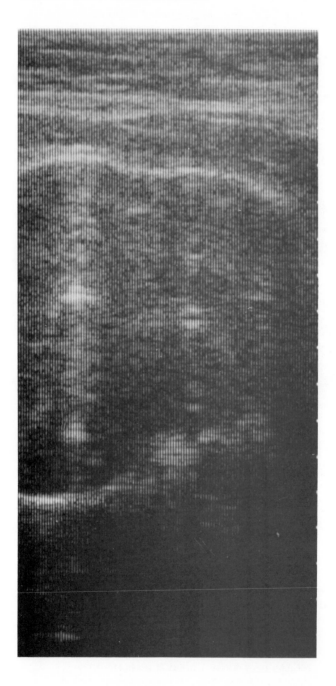

but can be suspected by ultrasound when the cranial outline is elongated and the contour uneven. Sometimes the cranial configuration can be mistaken for a cranial abnormality such as an encephalocele, especially when the head is wedged deep in the pelvis (Figures 3a and 3b).

Multiple gestations

A collaborative study of 6,503 sets of twins delivered at 32 different hospitals between 1961 and 1972 has been published (16). The overall perinatal mortality rate in this series was 12.4%. When only those twins weighing more than 1,000 g were considered, the perinatal loss was 6.16%, which was approximately three times greater than that of comparable singletons at the same institutions. While prematurity is primarily responsible for the high perinatal mortality in twins, they also have an increased incidence of congenital anomalies, placenta previa, abruptio placenta, toxemia, cord accidents, and malpresentations. Twins are at greatly increased risk of developing obstetrical problems, and the problems are augmented in the case of triplets and quadruplets. The intelligent use of ultrasound in the management of multiple gestations should help reduce the perinatal loss in this group.

Diagnosis and development

A widely quoted statistic is that about 50% of twins remain undiagnosed until the time of delivery (6, 9). This figure is probably now excessive because of the widespread utilization of ultrasound during the antenatal period in North America. The trend toward earlier diagnosis is encouraging because it increases the opportunity to offer specialized antenatal care. Multiple gestations should be suspected whenever the uterus seems to be larger than dates, when hydramnios or unexplained anemia develops, or when there is a suspicion that more than one fetal heart is being auscultated. Twins may be serendipitously diagnosed at the time of ultrasound scanning prior to a genetic amniocentesis or as a result of an elevated serum alphafetoprotein level in mass screening programs.

Individual normal twins grow at the same rate as singletons up to 30 or 32 weeks of gestation. Following this time, they do not gain weight as rapidly as singletons of the same gestational age (18). Daw and Walker (7) have stated that after 30 weeks the combined weight gain of the twins is approximately equivalent to that gained by a singleton for the remaining portion of the pregnancy. The reduction in each twin's somatic growth is believed to be due to the fact that at some point in the third trimester the placenta can no longer keep pace with the nutrient requirements of both developing fetuses, and this phenomenon occurs even earlier than 30 weeks when more than two fetuses are present. Interestingly, however, biparietal diameter (BPD) growth in two series of uncomplicated twin pregnancies has been shown to be similar to that of singleton fetuses of the same gestational age throughout the third trimester (14, 23). The disparity between normal BPD growth in the face of somatic deprivation is compatible with so-called "brain sparing," a mechanism whereby mildly growth-retarded infants preferentially favor head growth at the expense of increases in body weight.

In the large collaborative study cited above (16), 97% of twin sets weighed within 999 g. of each other at birth. In 18% of cases, however, the birth weights of each twin varied between 500 and 999 g. Obviously, this difference can be constitutional when the twins are dizygotic. There are, however, a number of pathological situations in which twins may be born with significant weight differences. These include the twin-to-twin transfusion syndrome, the combination of an anomalous fetus with a normal co-twin, and growth retardation affecting only one twin because of local placental factors.

The transfusion syndrome can only be present in monozygotic twins who share a monochorial placenta (Figure 4). The possibility of this syndrome occurs when the arterial circulation of one twin is in communication with the venous circulation of the other through arteriovenous shunts in the "common villous district" of a monochorial placenta (Figure 5) (1). In this situation one fetus becomes a donor who transfuses its co-twin. The donor becomes anemic and growth-retarded. Although, occasionally, it may become hydropic as a result of high outpatient failure, more frequently the donor is significantly smaller than the recipient (Figure 6). The recipient, on the other hand, becomes polycythemic and can go into congestive heart failure as a result of circulatory overload. It may also suffer thrombosis of peripheral vessels in association with its hypertransfused state. The perinatal mortality associated with the transfusion syndrome may be as high as 70% (1).

Significant congenital anomalies may occur in only one twin. Although it is conceivable that such an affected fetus might be normal in size, or hydropic with associated hydramnios, in most cases its growth lags significantly behind that of its normal co-twin. Finally, local factors can affect the placenta of only one twin.

Figure 4

Diagram of the two types of twin placentation. At the left is the
monochorionic (diamnionic) twin placenta, which is diagnostic of
monozygotic twinning, and at the right, a dichorionic placenta, which
is the placentation of all dizygotic twins; however, about 30% of
monozygotic twins have this mode of implantation also.

From Benirschke (1).

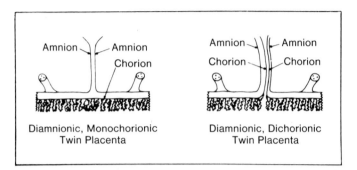

These include partial abruption, infarction, or unequal
allotment and development of placental areas. Growth
retardation of one twin due to inadequate placental
performance exposes that fetus to the same risks as
any singleton with IUGR.

When twins are differentially stressed in utero, it is
possible for one to die while the other continues to live
and grow. A maternal coagulopathy may develop as a
result of the release of thromboplastic material from the
retained dead fetus. An awareness of the intrauterine
demise of one twin permits the obstetrician to follow
weekly maternal clotting profiles and terminate the
pregnancy in the event that early evidence of
disseminated intravascular coagulation (DIC) develops.

The use of ultrasound

Separate gestational sacs can be identified
ultrasonically up to 10 weeks of gestational age (Figure
7). For the next 2 to 4 weeks the membranes
separating these sacs can almost always be seen, and
separate fetal bodies can be detected. Beyond 14
weeks fetal heads can easily be visualized and BPD's
measured. The ultrasonic diagnosis of multiple
gestations should, therefore, be quite straightforward.
Unfortunately, however, mistakes can be made
regarding the number of fetuses present when scans
are hastily performed. It must be remembered that an
ultrasound image, unlike a film of the abdomen, does
not display a composite overview. It only provides a
tomographic slice through the area being studied. It is,

Figure 5

Diagram of the placental vascular arrangement of the "transfusion syndrome" of monochorionic monozygotic twins. *A* is the smaller donor and *B* the plethoric recipient.

From Benirschke (1).

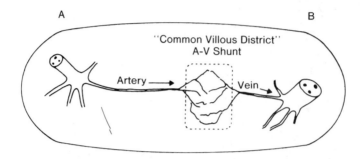

therefore, possible to visualize two circles that may represent different fetal heads or, alternatively, the head and thorax or abdomen of the same fetus in a tucked position (Figure 8). Only by unequivocally establishing the relationship of these circles to each other and to the remaining fetal parts can the actual number of fetuses be determined. An alternative problem that may occur if scanning is performed in a careless manner is the failure to observe a second fetus whose head is deeply engaged in the pelvis or pushed up under the ribs. The ultrasonographer must be compulsive in examining the entire intrauterine cavity. The scan should not be completed until the orientations of all the various fetal parts displayed are understood relative to each other (Figures 9 to 11).

Ultrasonic scanning on a regular basis permits an ongoing assessment of individual growth. Measurement of biparietal diameters is the most obvious method of identifying divergent growth patterns in twins. In a study by Houlton, 28 sets of twins had serial BPD measurements performed at either weekly or 2-week intervals (14). It was found that the rate of growth was similar in 39% of these cases and divergent in the remaining 61%. When the rates were divergent, the smaller BPD was always below the mean for singleton fetuses of similar gestational age. When the discrepancy in BPD's was between 2 and 6 mm, the incidence of low birth weight infants was 40%. When the difference was in excess of 6 mm, the incidence of low birth weight infants rose to 71%.

More sophisticated indices than the biparietal diameter

Figure 6

Twin-to-twin transfusion. Hydramnios is present, and the abdomen of
the twin on the right is significantly smaller than that on the left.
Notice that a rim of ascites is present in the abdomen of the larger
twin.

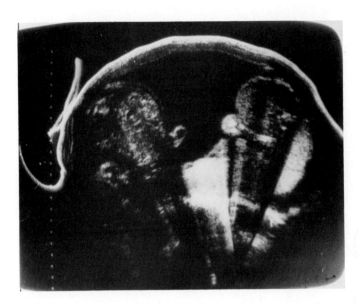

are available for assessing the developmental progress
of a fetus. Total intrauterine volume (TIUV) has been a
very valuable adjunct in the diagnosis of IUGR (10).
The TIUV is a measurement of the volume occupied by
all of the intrauterine contents, including the fetus, the
placenta, and the amniotic fluid. The published
nomogram, however, was derived from singleton
pregnancies. Unfortunately, it provides very little help in
diagnosing IUGR in twins because the TIUV in multiple
gestations is invariably several standard deviations
above the mean for singletons. The TIUV can be useful,
however, in estimating the amount of fluid that has
accumulated over 1-week intervals in twin pregnancies
when hydramnios has developed.

The biparietal diameter alone is a poor index of fetal
weight, but when BPD is utilized in association with the
abdominal circumference (AC) Shepard, et al. (24)
report estimated fetal weights that are more accurate.
In twin gestations measurement of both BPD's and
AC's can be technically quite difficult if one twin is lying
on top of the other. These measurements can often be
made, however, and when obtainable they are
extremely useful.

The head-to-body ratio is another index that has been

Figure 7

Fetal echoes visible in separate sacs of a twin gestation at 7 weeks.

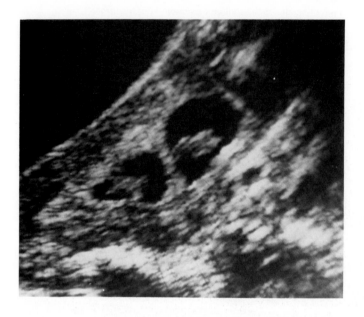

valuable in evaluating singleton fetuses for IUGR (5).
The AC is measured at the level of the umbilical
vein-portal sinus confluence and the head
circumference at the level of the biparietal diameter. In
general, after 36 weeks a normal fetus will have an
abdominal circumference larger than its head
circumference. Unfortunately, this is not particularly
helpful in twins because of the phenomenon of head
sparing.

Ultrasound during labor and delivery

An in-depth discussion of the management of twin
pregnancies during labor and delivery is not relevant to
this book. However, there are two ways in which
ultrasound can be of assistance in the delivery suite.

There is little question that if a patient with twins is
permitted to deliver vaginally both fetuses should be
monitored throughout labor (2). If membranes are
ruptured, a scalp clip can be applied to the vertex of
twin A and a Doppler belt used to monitor twin B. At
Yale-New Haven Hospital, if the presenting twin is in a
breech presentation the patient is delivered by
cesarean section. If twin A is in a vertex presentation
but membranes are not ruptured, it is possible to
monitor both twins with external belts. Obviously,
monitoring both twins requires the use of two fetal
monitors. Real-time ultrasound is very useful in locating

Figure 8

Two circles visible on a B-mode scan. Further scanning is necessary in order to identify the structures they represent. Five years ago this was a problem.

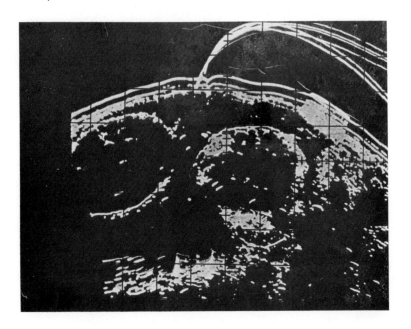

the optimal position to place a Doppler monitoring belt for each of the twins. The obstetrician can then be absolutely certain that both fetuses are being accurately monitored. A technique has been described that permits the uterine contraction pattern derived from an internal catheter to be displayed on two monitors simultaneously (6, 22). If one monitor is placed on top of the other, however, the contraction pattern registering on one can be visually transferred to the second tracing without difficulty.

A second use for real-time ultrasonography occurs at the time of vaginal delivery. After the first twin has been delivered, rapid real-time assessment can accurately delineate the position of twin B. If an internal version is necessary for the second twin, the lower extremities can be easily located and the operator guided in his attempts to grab them. The operator's hand can be visualized on the real-time display and intrauterine manipulations observed during an internal version. At Yale-New Haven Hospital the real-time machine is routinely brought to the delivery room when twins are delivered vaginally, and we have found that an experienced ultrasonographer can greatly assist with the delivery of the second twin.

Figure 9

Two perfect BPD's in a twin gestation. Notice the membranes separating the two sacs.

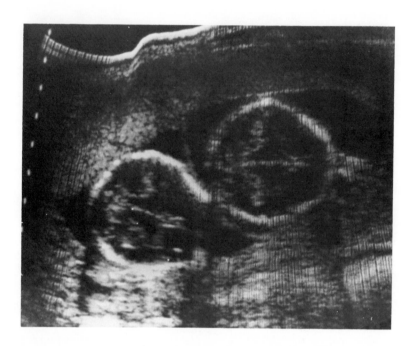

Recommendations

Patients should be sent for ultrasound examination if uterine size seems to be incompatible with dates. The earlier this is done the better. If a multiple gestation is diagnosed, the patient can be followed with serial examinations to be sure that development is progressing normally. If, on the other hand, the discrepancy is due to incorrect dating, gestational age can most accurately be determined ultrasonically by an examination prior to 26 weeks.

Amniocentesis for genetic diagnostic purposes should always be preceded by ultrasonic evaluation. This not only aids in selecting an insertion site for the needle but also provides accurate dates for the pregnancy as well as an opportunity to diagnose a multiple gestation. Once twins have been detected in this setting, it is strongly recommended that the patient be sent home to consider the implications of that diagnosis for subsequent genetic studies. This subject, as well as a description of the technique for performing amniocentesis in twins, is discussed in detail in Chapter 8.

When a multiple gestation has been diagnosed, the

Figure 10
> Transverse scan through the abdomens of a set of twins at 33 weeks.
> Numerous fetal limbs are evident in cross section.

From Berkowitz, R.L.: Ultrasound in the Antenatal Management of Multiple
Gestations. Clin. Diagn. Ultrasound 3:69, 1979.

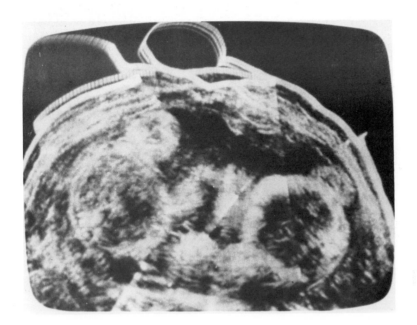

patient should be scanned every 4 weeks to measure
BPD and TIUV. This should be continued as long as no
hydramnios develops and the cranial measurements
remain within 2 mm of each other. Should excess fluid
accumulate or the growth of the BPD's become
divergent, more frequent ultrasonic assessments are
recommended.

Amniocentesis for genetic or ΔOD_{450} studies should be
performed on each twin sac. L/S ratios may be
performed on only one sac if both twins are equal in
size. If one twin is smaller than the other, however, the
possibility of differential stress in utero should be
considered, and, if possible, both sacs should be
tapped for L/S ratio determinations. If only one sac is
to be tapped in this setting, it should be the sac of the
twin that appears to be normal, as the stressed twin
can be assumed to have an L/S ratio which is at least
as mature as its normal counterpart and probably more
so.

Real-time ultrasound can be very useful on the labor
floor by locating the sites for appropriate placement of
external fetal heart rate monitoring belts. When taken

Figure 11

Sagittal scan of a twin gestation with separate anterior and posterior placentas. The membrane separating these sacs is easily seen.

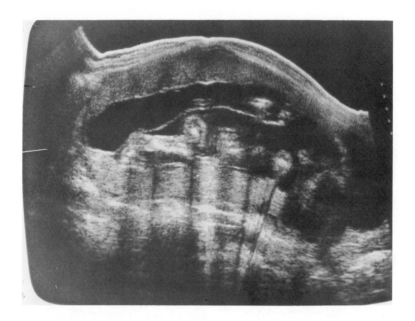

to the delivery room, real-time units permit accurate determination of the lie of twin B and greatly facilitate the performance of an internal version for the second twin should this become necessary.

Diabetes

Fifteen years ago the perinatal mortality rate (PNMR) in diabetes approached 50%. Today the PNMR in well-controlled diabetics is similar to that of non-diabetics. Many factors are responsible for this remarkable improvement in fetal salvage, but the most significant are attention to scrupulous diabetic control and better methods to assess fetal condition.

Diabetes affects the fetus and placenta in various ways that can be appreciated by ultrasound if the observer is sensitive to them. A thorough ultrasound evaluation of the pregnant diabetic encompasses many of the points elsewhere in this book.

Dating

Since timing of evaluation procedures scheduled for the pregnant diabetic is based on gestational age, it is necessary to date the pregnancy precisely with ultrasound. Relying upon the last menstrual period (LMP) in diabetic women is especially hazardous because they are often oligoamenorrheic. As in uncomplicated pregnancies, the earlier the scan, the more accurate the estimation of gestational age.

Crown-rump measurements

Today diabetics are counseled by their physicians to register as soon as they suspect they are pregnant, allowing pregnancy dating in the first trimester. Pederson found that crown-rump lengths were on an average 5.4 days smaller than those in non-diabetics of the same age (21). Since this finding is surprising in view of the tendency for insulin-dependent diabetics to deliver macrosomic fetuses, these results must be confirmed by other studies. As discussed in a previous chapter, crown-rump length is perhaps the most precise way to document gestational age, and should be attempted in diabetics who seek medical care in the first trimester.

BPD

As stated earlier, crown-rump length becomes an imprecise tool to assess gestational age after the 12th week, so one must resort to the BPD. In diabetics it is even more important to obtain BPD measurements as early as possible in pregnancy since fetal macrosomia is a feature of gestational (class A) and insulin-dependent diabetics without coagulopathy (class B and C). IUGR often complicates the pregnancies of diabetics with end organ disease (class D, F, R). In the former case BPD's tend to be above the mean in late gestation, and in the latter situation the BPD's often fall below the mean.

Various studies have demonstrated BPD's in diabetics to be either larger than average, less than average, or not different from non-diabetics. These apparent discrepancies can be explained by examining the study patients by class. If the BPD curve is heavily weighted with class D, F, and R diabetics, then BPD's tend to be smaller. On the other hand, if there is a liberal sampling of poorly controlled class A and B diabetics, the BPD average would suggest large-for-dates heads. Since the merits of tight diabetic control have been recognized, and because head size is less affected than that of the body in minimal macrosomia, we have found that the BPD's tend to be near the mean in well-controlled diabetics.

Amniotic fluid

Diabetics may accumulate more amniotic fluid than non-diabetics in late pregnancy. This is reflected in somewhat elevated TIUV values for dates. However, the TIUV is rarely more than 1 S.D. above the mean for

Figure 12

Sagittal scan of a macrosomic fetus in vertex presentation at 32 weeks.

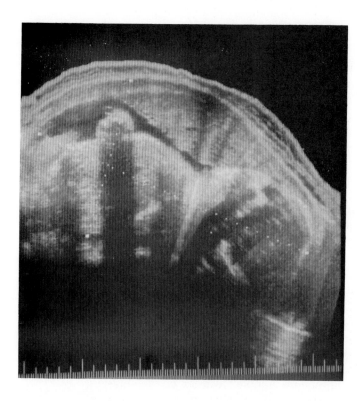

gestation, a quantity insufficient to be considered polyhydramnios. True polyhydramnios can occur in diabetics but should alert the physician to the possibility of a fetal anomaly.

One author (20) has reported that urine production rates in fetuses of the diabetic he studied were no different than those of fetuses of the same gestational age in non-diabetics. Nevertheless, we have observed that the fetal bladder in diabetics often appears unusually large and, anecdotally, the poorer the diabetic control, the greater the amount of amniotic fluid. On occasion the finding of a large fetal bladder has alerted us to the presence of glucose intolerance in previously undiagnosed gestational diabetics.

Head-to-body ratios

We have recently found that the more macrosomic the fetus of a diabetic the greater the body-to-head disproportion as measured by the ratio of head-to-abdominal circumference (Figure 12). This observation is consistent with the results from a study by Ogata et al. (19) in which they found BPD unreliable in identifying macrosomia but abdominal circumference to be larger than the mean in all of 10 macrosomic fetuses of diabetic mothers. Under the influence of fetal insulin released in response to hyperglycemia, increased quantities of triglycerides are incorporated into the fetal subcutaneous tissues. In addition, the liver of some fetuses of diabetics is huge. Growth of the body in excess of cranial enlargement may result in head-to-body ratios that are in the 5th percentile. Such disproportion should suggest the possibility of shoulder dystocia in a large fetus, since the growth hormone-like potential of fetal insulin also affects the shoulder girth.

Growth-retarded fetuses born to diabetics with renal or retinal vascular disease usually display head-to-body disproportion resulting from asymmetrical IUGR. If, however, placental compromise occurs early in gestation, these growth-retarded fetuses may have a head-to-body ratio within normal limits. Therefore, in diabetics, the estimation of both fetal weight and head-to-body ratio is far more useful than either measurement alone.

Fetal weight

Formulae using multiple fetal dimensions are more precise in predicting fetal weight than methods using only one dimension. This is especially true in diabetics in whom relative body and head proportions vary from the norm. Although the percent error is the same for all weight ranges, the absolute error predicted by the formula of Shepard et al. is greater for large fetuses than for those which are very small. Nevertheless, these estimated fetal weights (EFW) are invaluable when planning labor management for diabetics. If we calculate the EFW to be more than 4000 g and the head-to-body ratio indicates significant body-to-head disproportion, the patient will be delivered by cesarean section rather than risking infant morbidity from a traumatic vaginal delivery.

Placenta

The placenta is not immune to the growth-enhancing effects of fetal insulin, and, therefore, the placentas of macrosomic fetuses can become significantly enlarged (Figure 13). One should suspect an enlarged placenta when the thickness is more than 5 cm in sections obtained at right angles to its long axis. If excessive amounts of amniotic fluid are present, this finding may not be apparent because the placenta can become stretched out over an expanded uterus. In diabetics with growth-retarded fetuses, on the other hand, the placentas may be small.

Figure 13

Placental hypertrophy associated with fetal macrosomia in a diabetic pregnancy.

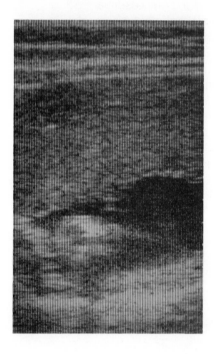

In diabetics it is useful to evaluate placental morphology. Grade 0 placentas are rarely noted after 30 weeks in normal pregnancies, except in gestational diabetes. The detection of a grade 0 placenta after 30 weeks should suggest the possibility of unsuspected glucose intolerance. In diabetics with compromised placental function, grade 3 placentas may be seen prior to 36 weeks. This is especially true if IUGR or hypertension complicates the pregnancy.

Fetal anomalies

Diabetics have a six times greater chance of delivering a baby with a major congenital abnormality. There are data suggesting, however, that good diabetic control in the first trimester will be associated with a major reduction in fetal anomalies.

The most common fetal abnormalities in diabetics involve the heart and include interventricular septal defects, hypoplastic ventricles, transposition of the great vessels, and atretic valves. It is possible with fetal echocardiography to identify many of these cardiac defects by the 24th week of gestation (15). Other anomalies common to the diabetic are neural tube defects, ventral wall defects, and intestinal obstruction. Caudal agenesis, the one defect which seems to be specific for infants of diabetic mothers, is fortunately quite rare. In view of the high incidence of fetal anomalies in diabetes we recommend that when the pregnancy is initially dated, particular attention be directed to a search for common anomalies. If, for example, a lethal condition such as anencephaly is found, the pregnancy can be terminated promptly without subjecting the patient to further diabetogenic stresses of pregnancy. Also, surgically correctable lesions, such as duodenal atresia or gastroschisis, can be identified early so that obstetrical management can be adjusted to include timely delivery in a hospital capable of providing the personnel and equipment for appropriate corrective measures.

Fetal echocardiography can provide important information concerning the status of the fetus of a diabetic. We have recently noted that the thickness of the interventricular septum is an indirect index of the quality of diabetic control. In some patients who sustain high blood sugars the septum is unusually thick. When blood sugars are lowered the septum returns to normal dimension within a few weeks. Macrosomic fetuses have large hearts. However, the septal hypertrophy seen in hyperglycemic fetuses is significantly larger than the other cardiac dimensions (4, 11).

Rh disease

The introduction of Rh (D) immune globulin (Rh IG) in 1968 has dramatically reduced the incidence of Rh hemolytic disease. Unfortunately, it has not eliminated the condition entirely, and women who are already sensitized will continue to become pregnant. Reasons for the appearance of new cases of Rh immunization include failure to administer Rh IG to all candidates following delivery, abortion, version, or amniocentesis; refusal of some candidates to accept prophylactic treatment for religious reasons; failure to give adequate quantities of Rh IG following massive feto-maternal hemorrhages; sensitization prior to delivery in the second and third trimesters; and mismatched blood transfusions. Furthermore, sensitization to atypical red cell antibodies is not affected by the administration of Rh IG. Therefore, despite the existence of Rh IG, a small but stable number of sensitized women with fetuses at risk for erythroblastosis fetalis will continue to present themselves for obstetric care.

Monitoring of serum titers of maternal antibodies is a notoriously inaccurate way to follow the progress of a sensitized woman's fetus. Studies of amniotic fluid offer

Figure 14

Liley graph of ΔOD$_{450}$ vs. gestational age.

From Frigoletto, F.D., Umanski, I.: Erythroblastosis fetalis: A basis for practice and prevention. In *Perinatal Medicine in Primary Practice*, J.B. Warshaw, J.C. Hobbins, eds. Addison-Wesley, Menlo Park, CA, 1982.

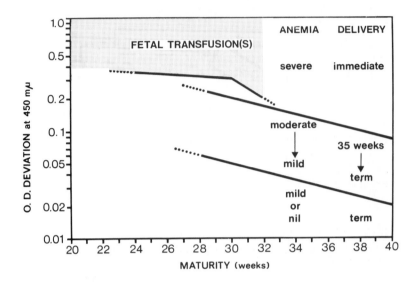

a more direct evaluation of fetal status. The most widely used assay is a simple photospectrometric analysis of fluid obtained at amniocentesis in order to measure the quantity of bilirubin pigment present. This determination is performed by measuring the deviation of the fluid sample at 450 mμ from the linear projection of the spectral absorption curve, and it is referred to as the ΔOD$_{450}$. By plotting serial ΔOD$_{450}$ values on a three-zoned graph designed by Liley, it is possible to evaluate the severity of fetal compromise (Figure 14) (17). Values in the lowest zone indicate that the fetus is unaffected or only minimally affected. Values in the upper zone indicate that the fetus is so severely affected that death is imminent unless it is transfused in utero or delivered and given an exchange transfusion. The middle zone is equivocal and requires follow-up.

A number of investigators have described modifications of this method for assessing the severity of erythroblastosis. Some have utilized techniques other than spectrophotometry to measure the quantity of bilirubin in amniotic fluid. None of these alternative approaches, however, has been shown to be conclusively superior to simple spectrophotometry and the use of the Liley graph if uncontaminated fluid is obtained at the time of amniocentesis. Blood,

Figure 15

Hydrops fetalis secondary to erythroblastosis fetalis. Notice the enlarged, fluffy placenta, fetal ascites, and edema of the abdominal wall.

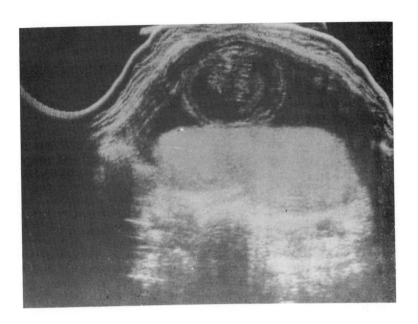

methemoglobin, and meconium in the fluid, however, can markedly interfere with the validity of readings at 450 mμ. Other sources of error include the inadvertent aspiration of fetal urine or ascitic fluid at the time of amniocentesis, or exposure of the amniotic fluid sample to light, which destroys bilirubin by photodegradation.

At Yale-New Haven Hospital, sensitized women who have indirect Coombs titers in excess of 1:8 or who have previously delivered affected children are followed with amniocentesis using simple spectrophotometry and the Liley graph. If a patient had a severely affected fetus in a preceding pregnancy, serial amniocenteses are begun at 20 to 21 weeks; otherwise they are initiated at 24 weeks. Once begun, amniotic fluid taps are performed every 2 weeks until delivery. If the values show an upward progression in the middle zone, taps are done weekly. When the ΔOD_{450} moves into the upper zone, the fetus is either transfused in utero or delivered within 24 hrs.

At the time of each amniocentesis, a thorough ultrasonic evaluation of the placenta or fetus should be made to look for evidence of hemolytic disease. When a sensitized fetus becomes hydropic, polyhydramnios is often present. Classic ultrasound findings include a thickened edematous placenta (Figure 15), generalized fetal edema (particularly evident over the scalp), and ascites. An early sign of incipient hydrops may be a demonstrable increase in the diameter of the umbilical vein, measured either within the hepatic parenchyma or in loops of cord floating freely in the amniotic fluid (8). While it is usually true that abnormalities in the ΔOD_{450} values are detected before ultrasonically evident signs of hydrops are present, this is not always the case. We have seen a Kell-sensitized patient in whom fetal hydrops and death in utero occurred prior to a significant elevation in ΔOD_{450} (3). It is, therefore, necessary that a thorough ultrasound evaluation be performed at the time of each amniocentesis for ΔOD_{450} determination.

Premature labor

In an effort to improve neonatal salvage, patients in premature labor are now referred to institutions with newborn special care units. Since there is some morbidity associated with administration of labor-inhibiting agents, protocols have been designed to select only those patients who clearly need them. For example, a patient whose fetus is more than 35 weeks should be excluded from treatment. However, since the patient's dates are misleading or unknown in almost 30% of cases, ultrasound estimation of gestational age is required in premature labor. The notoriously poor correlation between BPD and gestational age in late gestation has been repeatedly stated. However, in this clinical setting the BPD, along with measurements of abdominal circumference at the level of the umbilical vein-portal sinus anastomosis and femur length, can be helpful in validating the patient's dates.

Sometimes patients in labor are referred to tertiary care hospitals very early in their pregnancies. If attempts to stop labor are unsuccessful, the physician must quickly assess the chances of survival of the fetus in the event of fetal distress. The salvage rates of premature babies vary between institutions, and it is important for those in each referral facility to review newborn statistics periodically in an effort to develop survival probabilities for different birth weights (or gestational ages). At Yale-New Haven Hospital in 1980 there was about a 60% chance of survival if the infant weighed between 700 and 1000 g. If, on the other hand, the infant weighed less than 650 g, there were no survivors who were not hopelessly brain-damaged. Ultrasound should, therefore, play a key role in decision making regarding the management of premature labor.

Hypertension is a frequently encountered condition in pregnancy, and ultrasound is helpful in its management. Placental texture, as described in Chapter 4, may be a clue to stress in utero related to maternal hypertension. However, ultrasound's greatest contribution in this condition is the diagnosis of IUGR, a subject covered in Chapter 6.

Other examples of how ultrasonically derived information can aid in obstetrical management include monitoring the size and location of suprapubic fibroids or the status of a kidney transplant. In the former case one can assess the chances of vaginal delivery before subjecting the patient to a long labor. In the latter case it is possible to observe the extent of compression of the implanted kidney. Even though many infants have been delivered vaginally by patients with renal transplants, there are some women in whom the risks of vaginal delivery are not warranted if significant kidney compression is noted in early labor.

References

1 **Benirschke, K., Kim, C.K.**: Multiple pregnancy. N. Engl. J. Med. 288:1276, 1973.

2 **Berkowitz, R.L.**: The antenatal assessment and management of twin gestations. Perinatal Care 2:28, 1978.

3 **Berkowitz, R.L., Beyth, Y., Sadovsky, E.**: Death in utero due to Kell-sensitization without excessive elevation of the ΔOD_{450} value in amniotic fluid. Obstet. Gynecol., in press.

4 **Breitweser, J.A., Meyer, R.A., Sperling, M.A., Tsang, R.C., Kaplan, S.**: Cardiac septal hypertrophy in hyperinsulinemic infants. J. Pediatr. 96:535, 1980.

5 **Campbell, S., Thoms, A.**: Ultrasound measurement of the fetal head-to-abdomen circumference ratio in assessment of growth retardation. Br. J. Obstet. Gynaecol. 84:165, 1977.

6 **Centrulo, C.L., Freeman, R.K., Knuppel, R.A.**: Minimizing the risk of twin delivery. Contemp. Ob/Gyn 9:2:47, 1977.

7 **Daw, E., Walker, J.**: Growth differences in twin pregnancy. Br. J. Clin. Practice 29:150, 1975.

8 **DeVore, G.R., Mayden, K., Tortora, M., Berkowitz, R.L., Hobbins, J.C.**: Dilation of the fetal umbilical vein in rhesus hemolytic anemia: A predictor of severe disease. Am. J. Obstet. Gynecol. 141:464, 1981.

9 **Farooqui, M.O., Grossman, J.H., III, Shannon, R.A.**: A review of twin pregnancy and perinatal mortality. Obstet. Gynecol. Surv. (Suppl.) 28:144, 1973.

10 **Gohari, P., Berkowitz, R.L., Hobbins, J.C.**: Prediction of intrauterine growth retardation by determination of total intrauterine volume. Am. J. Obstet. Gynecol. 127:255, 1977.

11 **Gutgesell, H.P., Speer, M.E., Rosenberg, H.S.**: Characterization of

the cardiomyopathy in infants of diabetic mothers. Circulation 61:2, 441, 1980.

12 **Hadlock, F.P., Deter, R.L., Carpenter, R.J., Park, S.K.**: Estimating fetal age: Effect of head shape on BPD. Am. J. Roentgenol. Radium Ther. Nucl. Med. 137:83, 1981.

13 **Hobbins, J.C.**: Use of ultrasound in critical decisions in obstetrical management. In *Diagnostic Ultrasound Applied to Obstetrics and Gynecology*, R.E. Sabbagha, ed. Harper and Row, New York, 1980.

14 **Houlton, M.C.C.**: Divergent biparietal diameter growth rates in twin pregnancies. Obstet. Gynecol. 49:542, 1977.

15 **Kleinman, C.S., Hobbins, J.C., Jaffe, C.C., Lynch, D.C., Talner, N.S.**: Echocardiographic studies of the developing human fetus: Prenatal diagnosis of congenital heart disease and cardiac dysrhythmias. Pediatrics 65:6, 1059, 1980.

16 **Kohl, S.G., Casey, G.**: Twin gestation. Mt. Sinai J. Med. 42:523, 1975.

17 **Liley, A.W.**: Liquor amnii analysis in the management of the pregnancy complicated by rhesus sensitization. Am. J. Obstet. Gynecol. 82:1359, 1961.

18 **McKeown, T., Record, R.G.**: Observations on foetal growth in multiple pregnancy in man. J. Endocrinol. 8:386, 1952.

19 **Ogata, E.S., Sabbagha, R., Metzger, B.E., Phelps, R.L., Depp, R., Freinkel, N.**: Serial ultrasonography to assess evolving fetal macrosomia. J.A.M.A. 243:2405, 1980.

20 **Otterlo, L.C., Van Wladimiroff, J.W., Wallenburg, H.C.S.**: Relationship between fetal urine production and amniotic fluid volume in normal pregnancy and pregnancy complicated by diabetes. Br. J. Obstet. Gynaecol. 84:205, 1977.

21 **Pederson, J.F., Mølsted-Pedersen, L.**: Early fetal growth retardation in diabetic pregnancy. Br. Med. J. 6155:18, 1979.

22 **Read, J.A., Miller, F.C.**: Technique of simultaneous direct intrauterine pressure recording for electronic monitoring of twin gestation in labor. Am. J. Obstet. Gynecol. 129:228, 1977.

23 **Scheer, K.**: Ultrasound in twin gestation. J. Clin. Ultrasound 2:197, 1974.

24 **Shepard, M.J., Richards, V.M., Berkowitz, R.L., Warsof, S., Hobbins, J.C.**: An evaluation of two equations for predicting fetal weight by ultrasound. Am. J. Obstet. Gynecol. 142:47, 1982.

Intrauterine Growth Retardation

6

Intrauterine growth retardation (IUGR) is defined as a process that results in the birth of a neonate whose weight is below the 10th percentile for gestational age. These "small-for-gestational-age" (SGA) babies suffer from greatly increased perinatal morbidity and mortality and may have continuing developmental impairment when compared to "appropriate-for-gestational-age" (AGA) neonates. It is obvious that in order to reduce damage done by IUGR, the condition must be diagnosed as early as possible in utero rather than at birth.

Etiology

Intrauterine growth retardation is a non-specific term comprising a variety of developmental problems. Its two principal causes are inadequate supply of nutrients or oxygen, and decreased intrinsic growth potential of the fetus.

The former cause is more prevalent than the latter. Deficient nutrient or oxygen supply may be due to relative hypoxia in women who are anemic, have heart disease, or live at high altitude. It may also be associated with smoking, maternal malnutrition, and multiple gestations. Any maternal disorder that reduces blood flow to the intervillous space may result in "supply line" defects in fetal growth. These conditions include hypertension, chronic renal disease, severe diabetes with vascular involvement, and others which are less common (10). Primary placental causes include chronic partial separation, extensive infarction, and placenta previa.

Fetal abnormalities can be caused by genetic factors, exposure to teratogens, or infectious agents such as rubella, cytomegalic virus, or toxoplasmosis. Any of these may result in a primary reduction of fetal growth potential in addition to specific morphological malformations. Drugs, chemical compounds, or x-ray exposure may be teratogenic in the first trimester. A variety of congenital abnormalities can be associated with IUGR. Specific conditions in which this association has been observed include Potter, Turner, and Down syndromes, trisomy 18, and anencephaly.

In a Canadian study (21) published in 1974, 182 of 3428 consecutive deliveries (5.3%) resulted in SGA neonates. Only 95 (52%) of the patients with growth-retarded infants had predictive clues which put them at risk for developing this condition. Slightly less than half of these women had "high risk" indicators at the onset of their pregnancies, including a history of a prior perinatal death, recurrent abortions, or birth of an SGA infant. The remainder of these 95 women were recognized later in their pregnancies because of findings or complications such as multiple gestation, antenatally detected congenital abnormalities, postdatism, antepartum bleeding, and pre-eclampsia. The other 87 women who delivered SGA infants were believed to have had uncomplicated obstetrical courses. They could only have been detected if it had been appreciated that the fetus was too small for gestational age.

The growth-retarded neonate

A consideration of the appearance and metabolic problems of SGA neonates is useful in understanding the altered anatomy and physiology of growth-retarded fetuses. This, in turn, should provide clues for the ultrasonographer in diagnosing this condition in utero.

Appearance at Birth

Fifty percent of SGA babies show obvious soft tissue and muscle mass wasting at birth (Figure 1). This is particularly evident in the cheeks, arms, buttocks, and thighs. The skin may be dried and cracked with peeling over the palms and soles. The skull contour may be widened, but the fontanelles remain flat, suggesting diminished bone growth rather than increased intracranial pressure. These neonates are often vigorous and active at birth but can become depressed and lethargic as a result of antepartum asphyxia, persisting acidosis, or hypoglycemia.

Postpartum problems

SGA infants are at higher risk for perinatal asphyxia than those whose weight is appropriate for gestational age. Intrapartum asphyxia may lead to meconium aspiration leading to pneumonia, pneumothorax, and pulmonary hypertension. Metabolic acidosis secondary to asphyxia results in a compensatory respiratory alkalosis. This, in turn, can cause significant electrolyte imbalance with subsequent cerebral edema and convulsions. Growth-retarded neonates may be symptomatically polycythemic and suffer from

Figure 1

Growth-retarded newborn with obvious subcutaneous wasting. The placenta is abnormally small.

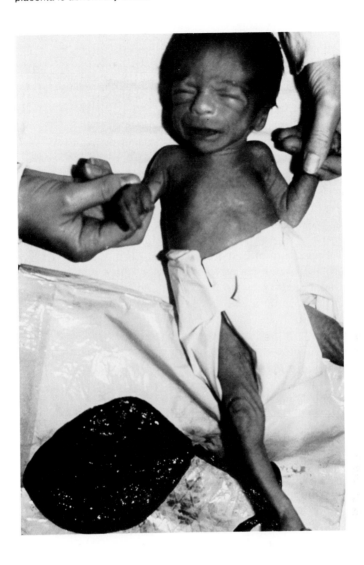

symptoms of hyperviscosity such as lethargy, irritability, seizures, and decreased renal function. The polycythemia may be due to intrauterine hypoxia or to placental-to-fetal transfusion at the time of hypoxic insult (33). Because of decreased subcutaneous fat and relatively large surface area for body weight, the SGA infant often has trouble maintaining body temperature.

Growth-retarded neonates have deficient subcutaneous and deep body fat that may restrict the postnatal development of fatty acid oxygenation by heart, brain, and other tissues. Decreased hepatic glycogen stores and deficient gluconeogenesis often contribute to symptomatic hypoglycemia. Significant muscle mass depletion can also result in a reduction in protein reserves.

The British Perinatal Mortality Survey (3) showed that among growth-retarded babies born after 36 weeks' gestation the number of intrapartum and neonatal deaths was almost eight times higher than for babies of similar age whose weight was appropriate. Usher and McLean (32) examined the perinatal morbidity figures in a series of 44,256 consecutive births over a 13-year period and found them 10 times as frequent in IUGR infants. They estimated that in their series 2.7 perinatal deaths per 1000 births were exclusively caused by chronic fetal nutritional deprivation.

Fitzhardinge and Steven (12) followed 96 full-term SGA infants for a minimum of 5 years from their birth. While major neurological defects were uncommon, there was an increased incidence of hyperactivity, short attention span, poor fine coordination, and school performance. The average IQ of the study group was very close to normal, but the authors conclude that they showed evidence of impaired development when compared with controls who were AGA at birth.

Fetal growth patterns

It has been widely accepted that human growth in utero resembles that of organisms in a limited environment where growth diminishes as nutritive supplies are exhausted. Fetal growth curves in which birth weight is plotted against gestational age at birth show progressively earlier deceleration in growth when twins are compared to singletons, triplets to twins, etc. Differences in third trimester "plateauing" have also been shown in different ethnic and socio-economic groups as well as in smokers when compared to non-smokers. However, Wilcox (36) has recently suggested that fundamental concepts underlying the formulation of these growth curves may be fallacious and suggests that growth in utero might be better followed by considering bivariate distributions of weight and age. Birnholz (2), using four or more serial ultrasonically derived estimated fetal weights, has calculated growth curves for several normal and growth-retarded fetuses. In the normal cases a near linear increase in weight was noted throughout the third trimester, and Birnholz believes that the decremental pattern observed in birth weight surveys may be due to statistical artifacts. He also points out that weight growth in the newborn is nearly linear at a rate identical to this third trimester average.

Martinez and Barton (24) have published nomograms for fetal body volume (FBV) and fetal head volumes (FHV) from 18 to 41 weeks of gestation. The FBV data are based on 198 observations and FHV on 317 observations in women who delivered AGA neonates. Least squares regression analysis of the data shows that mean FHV increases through gestation in a pattern approximating a straight line, while mean FBV increases in a pattern approximating a geometric growth function, i.e., the log of FBV is linearly related to the log of gestational age.

These considerations indicate that normal human growth in utero is incompletely understood, and cross-sectional data based on birth weight at different gestational ages may not reflect dynamic changes within a specific pregnancy. As our ability to accurately follow growth in utero increases, a parallel increase in understanding normal as well as abnormal patterns should evolve.

Winick et al. (37) have described two patterns of IUGR that can be experimentally induced in rats. When the mother is nutritionally deprived, the offspring are symmetrically small and DNA analysis of the brain reveals a decrease in both cell size and number. On the other hand, when uterine blood flow is mechanically compromised, there is asymmetrical fetal growth retardation with a significant reduction in the DNA content of the trunk and internal organs, whereas the brain is much less severely affected. These authors hypothesize that relative sparing of the head is due to preferential carotid vasodilatation in response to fetal hypoxia.

Campbell's (4) serial cephalometric studies have confirmed that the two different patterns of growth retardation observed in animal models also occur in humans. In "late flattening" IUGR, a diminution in the growth rate of the fetal head is first observed late in the third trimester. When delivered, these neonates are asymmetrical with small bodies and relatively normal-sized heads. Campbell found that this type of IUGR accounted for approximately 75% of the cases in his series and was frequently associated with conditions in which there is reduced placental perfusion. These infants had a high incidence of perinatal asphyxia and neonatal hypoglycemia. In "low profile" growth retardation, on the other hand, diminished BPD growth may be observed early in the second trimester and it persists until delivery. These infants are symmetrically growth-retarded, often very small, occasionally anomalous, and as a rule do not suffer from perinatal asphyxia. In follow-up studies on 60 SGA babies, Fancourt et al. (11) found significantly lower developmental quotients on the Griffiths scales when the onset of IUGR occurred prior to 26 weeks.

It is now generally accepted that asymmetrical growth retardation is due to the preferential shunting of blood to the fetal brain in situations of inadequate placental passage of nutrients or oxygen. In theory, this phenomenon allows the head to grow and the brain to develop at the expense of optimal growth of fetal body mass. In symmetrical IUGR, however, there is either an intrinsic alteration in fetal growth potential, or fetal nutritional deprivation has become so severe that the protective mechanisms of "brain sparing" have been overwhelmed.

Assessment of fetal development

The cheapest and most readily available diagnostic method for estimating fetal size is abdominal palpation. Unfortunately, it is not a very sensitive tool with which to evaluate intrauterine development. Loeffler (20) found that while clinical predictions of fetal weight were within 458 g in 80% of estimates, this degree of accuracy was only attained in 43% of cases with weights less than 2270 g. Campbell (4) has reported that only 33 of 115 SGA babies delivered at Queen Charlotte's Hospital in 1970 were clinically recognized prior to delivery.

Ultrasound assessment of the intrauterine contents has given us the ability to measure structures that are related to fetal size. Investigators have used these data in a variety of ways in an attempt to detect altered growth in utero more precisely. The following parameters can be measured:

Biparietal diameter The criteria for obtaining accurate BPD's have been extensively discussed in earlier chapters. This variable is a reasonable predictor of fetal weight prior to 30 weeks because it accurately assesses gestational age during a period when there is a good correlation between weight and age. During the last 10 weeks of pregnancy, however, the relationship is much less constant, especially in cases of IUGR. Furthermore, after the 30th week of gestation it is impossible to assess fetal BPD growth accurately over a 2-week period since the mean increase of BPD is less than 4 mm whereas the standard error of measurement is ± 2 mm.

Head circumference This is measured in the same cross section as the biparietal diameter. An image must

Figure 2

Diagram of axial section through fetal skull at the level of the thalami. D_1 and D_2 represent the diameters used to calculate head circumference.

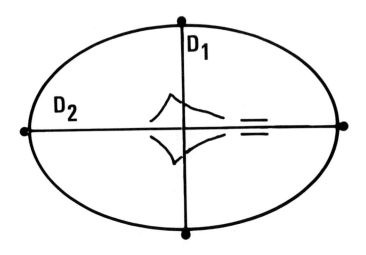

be obtained which cleanly displays at least 60 to 70% of the skull outline. The circumference may be measured either by running a map reader or electronic caliper around the outer margin of the skull table, or by measuring the largest sagittal (D_1) and transverse (D_2) diameters and then using the formula: $HC = ((D_1)/2 + (D_2)/2) \pi$ (Figure 2). When a map reader is used, the numbers on the dial must be converted to values which correspond to actual dimensions in utero. A conversion ratio is established by using the map reader to measure the distance between two points which are 10 cm apart on a graticule projected onto the scan. If, for example, this gives a reading of 8, a circumference which measures 24 on the map reader corresponds to an actual dimension of 30 cm (e.g., $8/10 = 24/\times$).

Head circumferences are no more accurate than BPD's in estimating fetal weights, but they can be compared to other fetal circumferential measurements when assessing developmental milestones.

Abdominal circumference An abdominal circumference (AC) measurement at the level of the umbilical vein has been shown to be a better predictor of fetal weight than the BPD. The appropriate level for obtaining this measurement is at right angles to the long axis of the fetus (verified by visualizing the length of the aorta) at the place where the umbilical vein branches into the portal sinus (Figure 3). The

Figure 3

Cross section of the fetal abdomen at the level of where the umbilical vein (*short arrow*) branches into the portal sinus (*long arrow*).

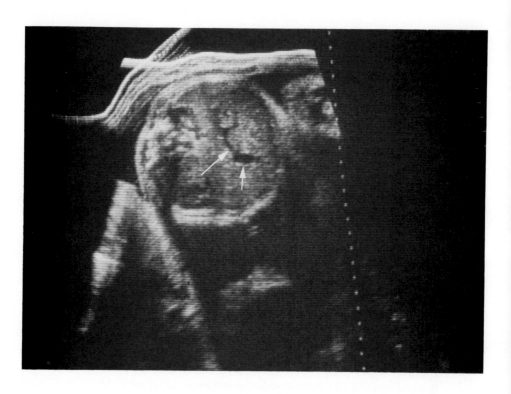

circumference should be almost circular if the transducer is properly oriented. An exaggerated oval circumference in the presence of normal amniotic fluid volume suggests that a tangential cut has been made through the fetal body. If the umbilical vein cannot be identified, the scan can be made at the level of the fetal stomach. Once an appropriate scanning cut has been achieved, the circumference is measured with a map reader, using the method described above, or by using the formula: $AC = ((D_1/2) + (D_2/2)) \pi$ (Figure 4).

Our group (9) and others (35) have demonstrated that abdominal circumference measurements obtained by linear arrays are not significantly different from those obtained by static scanners. Furthermore, in the other study, when the outline of the fetal AC was larger than the sonic field displayed by the array, the partially incomplete boundary could be "filled in" without affecting the accuracy of the result. When dynamic sector scanners are used, the outline is generally complete and extrapolation is unnecessary.

Chest circumference Some investigators have used

Figure 4

Diagram of cross section of fetal abdomen at the level of the umbilical vein branching into the portal sinus. D_1 and D_2 represent the diameters used to calculate the abdominal circumference.

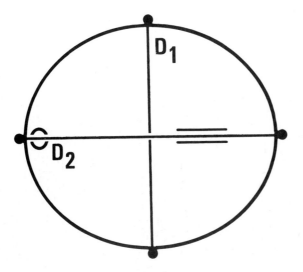

thoracic circumference or fetal chest area to assess fetal weight. These measurements should be made immediately caudal to the fetal heart pulsations. Again, efforts should be made to obtain a circular cut through the fetus at right angles to the thoracic vertebrae. Actual measurements are obtained in the same fashion described for the abdominal circumference.

Total intrauterine volume In the absence of compensatory changes, failure of any of the intrauterine components to grow properly should be reflected in the total intrauterine volume (TIUV). The TIUV can be computed by measuring the greatest longitudinal (L), transverse (T), and anteroposterior diameters (AP) of the uterus (Figures 5a and 5b) and then applying the following formula for calculating the volume of an ellipse (13):

$$V = 4/3 \, \pi \, (L/2 \times T/2 \times AP/2) = 0.5233 \times L \times T \times AP.$$

It is usually impossible to obtain the sagittal and transverse measurements necessary to calculate TIUV. with a real-time scanner in the third trimester. The transducer heads of currently available equipment are simply not long enough to permit visualization of these diameters in their entirety. It is, therefore, necessary to use an articulated static scanner when measuring most TIUV's after 26 to 28 weeks.

Figure 5a

Sagittal scans through the long axis of the uterus in two patients at 32 weeks of gestation. The scan on the *left* represents an appropriately grown fetus, while the one on the *right shows* a pregnancy with severe IUGR. Notice the "crowding" in utero which is obvious in the scan of the growth-retarded fetus. A small amount of amniotic fluid is present in the AGA fetus, while oligohydramnios is present in association with IUGR.

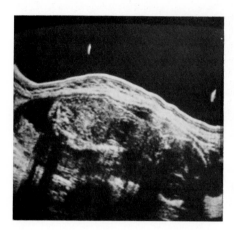 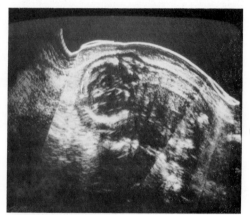

Fetal urine production The fetal bladder can be ultrasonically visualized and measured. Its volume can be determined by the same formula given for TIUV. By taking two sets of measurements 30 min. apart, the hourly fetal urine production rate (HFUPR) can be computed (8). If the bladder empties between the two examinations, a third study is required 30 min. later.

A nomogram has been published showing a steadily increasing HFUPR from 30 weeks to term (39). No circadian variation has been observed. In a series of 62 patients, 18 of 29 (62%) whose HFUPR was below the 5th percentile were growth-retarded at birth. Of the 22 SGA neonates in this series, 18 (82%) had HFUPR's below the normal range (39). This suggests that there is a significant correlation between IUGR and reduced fetal urine production. Unfortunately, this study is time-consuming and is technically difficult to perform so that it should still be regarded as a research tool.

Diagnosing IUGR

As defined at the beginning of this chapter, a fetus is considered to be growth-retarded if it is below the 10th percentile of weight for gestational age. A number of different approaches have been used in attempting to diagnose this condition in utero. Some have been indirect in that they have looked for sequelae of altered growth, while others have directly focused on attempting to accurately assess fetal weight.

Figure 5b

Transverse scans from the same two fetuses. Notice the normal amount of fluid on the *left* and the severe oligohydramnios on the *right*.

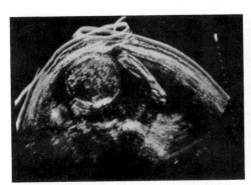
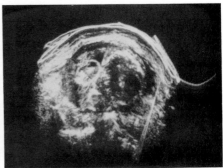

Indirect methods

BPD Campbell and Dewhurst (5) reported on a series of cases at risk for IUGR in which fetal growth was assessed with serial BPD measurements. When the growth rate of the BPD was below the 5th percentile, 82% (93 of 114) of the neonates were found to be below the 10th percentile of weight for gestational age. The other 18%, however, had birth weights within the normal range. On the other hand, 46 of 266 (17%) of babies whose BPD growth was within the normal range were below the 10th percentile of weight for gestational age at birth. The false-positive results (i.e., abnormally small BPD's in AGA infants) may have been due to errors inherent in third trimester cephalometry mentioned in earlier chapters. The false-negative results, however, were probably cases of asymmetrical IUGR where head involvement was minimal.

Sabbagha (29), using the method of GASA described in Chapter 3, found that 52% of fetuses with BPD's falling chronically below the 25th percentile and 20% of those with BPD's dropping to lower percentile ranks were growth-retarded. By contrast, the incidence of IUGR in fetuses whose BPD's were consistently above the 75th percentile or between the 25th and 75th percentiles was 3.5% and 10%, respectively.

While this may be more accurate than simply doing serial cephalometry in the third trimester, it still has a significant number of both false-positives and false-negatives, as will inevitably be true of any method relying exclusively on fetal head measurements that do not reflect growth retardation in a fetus with effective "brain sparing." It might be argued that when IUGR exists without any effect on fetal head size, the process has no significance for the fetus. This assumption, however, has not been proven and may well be false. Subtle central nervous system changes may precede a diminution in brain size, and long term effects on deprived organs in the chest and abdomen have not been studied. We, therefore, should strive to diagnose IUGR as early as possible, as this may have important therapeutic implications. Furthermore, it must be stressed that involvement of the head in asymmetrical IUGR indicates the chronicity of the process. Any method which relies on subnormal BPD growth to diagnose IUGR, therefore, cannot possibly pick up cases in which effective head sparing has occurred.

Head-to-abdomen ratio In asymmetrical growth retardation the ratio of head-to-body circumference is abnormal. In 1977 Campbell and Thoms (6) measured head and abdominal circumferences in 568 normal pregnancies between 17 and 41 weeks. They constructed a nomogram with 95% confidence limits that showed a mean head-to-abdomen (H:A) ratio of 1.18 at 17 weeks and a slow decrease to 1.11 at 29 weeks (see Appendix). Thereafter, there was a sharp fall in the mean ratio to 1:01 at 36 weeks and 0.96 at 40 weeks. In 31 SGA fetuses whose estimated fetal weights (EFW) were below the 5th percentile for gestation, the H:A ratio was above the 95th percentile in 71%. These infants were demonstrated to be asymmetrically growth-retarded at birth. The authors suggested, and others have confirmed, that the H:A ratio is an effective way to differentiate between symmetrical and asymmetrical growth retardation in utero.

Other potential uses for H:A ratios include the diagnoses of hydrocephaly and microcephaly, the evaluation of head-to-body disproportion in breeches being considered for vaginal delivery between 32 and 36 weeks, and the evaluation of an infant of a diabetic mother (IDM) for possible shoulder dystocia at term. In cases of poorly controlled diabetes there may be considerable body-to-head disproportion. Our studies have suggested that as fetal macrosomia increases in IDM's the head-to-body ratio decreases. If, therefore, the EFW exceeds 4000 g and the H:A ratio is below the 10th percentile, elective cesarean section should be considered in order to avoid a difficult vaginal delivery complicated by shoulder dystocia.

Head-to-chest ratio Wladimiroff et al. (38) have published a nomogram of fetal BPD-to-chest area ratios based on studies in 303 pregnancies which resulted in AGA neonates. In 84 documented cases of IUGR, the BPD was below the 5th percentile in 43% while the chest area was below the 5th percentile in 75%. The authors found that in this group of SGA infants a normal head-to-chest ratio was almost always associated with early onset of IUGR, while in the majority of fetuses with increased ratios the growth retardation was asymmetrical. This technique is based on the same principle underlying H:A studies. It offers no advantages over the latter and may be less accurate because of failure to make serial measurements at precisely the same level in the fetal chest. Other disadvantages include frequent shadowing of the chest by fetal upper extremities, and difficulty in following a thoracic wall outline that may be irregular in contour.

Total intrauterine volume By definition, fetal mass is reduced in IUGR. In addition, placental volume is invariably diminished and oligohydramnios is often present. It follows, therefore, that in the absence of unusual compensatory changes, the total intrauterine volume will reflect these reductions.

We have published a TIUV nomogram based on values obtained from 100 patients with uncomplicated pregnancies and BPD's compatible with their dates (Figure 6) (13). Ninety-six women were subsequently studied who were at risk of having a baby with IUGR or who were clinically suspected of having a growth-retarded fetus. Twenty-eight of the women delivered babies who were in or below the 10th percentile of weight for gestational age. The TIUV was more than 1½ standard deviations below the mean for 21 of these patients, and there were no normal pregnancies in this "abnormal zone." The remaining seven IUGR pregnancies had TIUV's which were between 1 and 1½ standard deviations below the mean. Because there were 15 normal pregnancies in the same range, this is referred to as the "gray zone." All of the remaining patients had AGA neonates and in each case their TIUV was less than 1 standard deviation below the mean.

Except for the cases which fell into the gray zone, the results were remarkably clear-cut. The seven IUGR neonates in the gray zone were, in fact, the most severely affected in the series. Two of these infants had congenital anomalies and three died. These patients fell into the gray zone because in each case the BPD lagged behind dates by more than 4 weeks and this was not appreciated. If the true dates had been known and used instead of those derived from the abnormally

Figure 6

Nomogram for TIUV showing division into normal, abnormal, and gray zones.

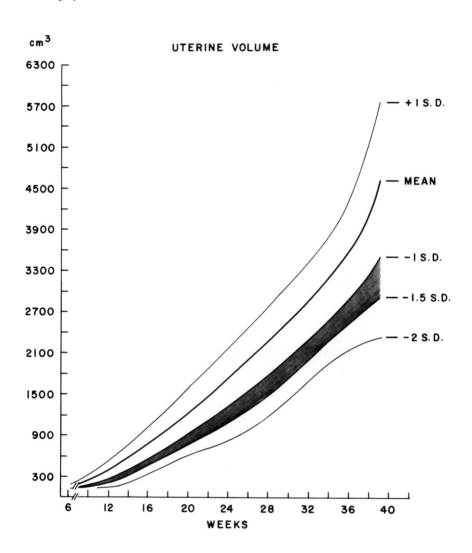

small BPD's, the TIUV's would all have been significantly more than 1-½ S.D.'s below the mean for gestations.

Since this initial study was published, we have used the TIUV in the evaluation of hundreds of pregnancies and continue to find it to be an extremely valuable tool in the assessment of a patient at risk for IUGR. The TIUV does not directly measure IUGR, but rather is a manifestation of its consequences. If it is abnormal, more sensitive indices of fetal size should be examined in order to make the diagnosis with greater precision. It is and must be thought of as a screening test.

While it is very rare for a growth-retarded fetus to have a normal TIUV, this could theoretically occur if placental hypertrophy or an increase in amniotic fluid volume were associated with a process which directly inhibited fetal growth potential. Occasionally AGA fetuses have TIUV's in the abnormal zone, but in these cases significant oligohydramnios is invariably present, for example, if the membranes are ruptured or in normal pregnancies at the extremes of a Gaussian distribution. In some cases no explanation for the oligohydramnios can be found and it is possible that in these instances the decrease in fluid is the first step in a process which, if allowed to continue, would result in IUGR.

Manning et al. (23) have capitalized on the usual association of oligohydramnios with IUGR in devising a screening test which is even simpler than measuring TIUV. They refer to their test as a qualitative amniotic fluid anywhere on the ultrasound scan measures at least 1 cm in its broadest diameter (Figure 7). In a series of 120 patients scanned to rule out IUGR, 91 were found to have normal AFV's. Eighty-six of these women (93.4%) delivered AGA neonates. On the other hand, 26 of 29 women with decreased qualitative AFV's (89.9%) delivered SGA babies. These data clearly indicate that IUGR is usually associated with a reduction in amniotic fluid. We feel, however, that although this method is easy to perform, it may be misleading in relatively unskilled hands. Collections of fluid may be difficult to visualize beneath a fetus in a heavy woman or when fetal parts and an anterior placenta create acoustic shadowing. Furthermore, while it is true that one usually sees pockets of fluid which fall within the "normal range" of this test, it does not correlate with any specific fluid volume. Despite the excellent results cited above, we are concerned about missing IUGR in cases where the AFV is normal. We have seen scans in which significant oligohydramnios was associated with growth retardation in patients having single pockets of amniotic fluid measuring more than 1 cm in depth.

We, therefore, prefer to measure the TIUV, since with a little more effort one is rewarded with a more quantitative parameter with which to follow the pregnancy. As already noted, however, TIUV's often cannot be measured with real-time scanners in the third trimester. When contact scanners are not available, the qualitative AFV may serve as a reasonable substitute for the TIUV as a screening test for IUGR.

Figure 7

This scan demonstrates a pocket of amniotic fluid with a depth of more than 1 cm. The two markers are 1 cm apart.

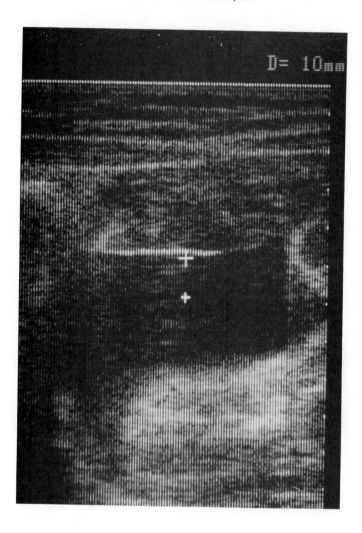

Direct methods

Accurate assessment of fetal weight is the key to the diagnosis of IUGR. If a fetus is below the 10th percentile for gestational age, it is growth-retarded according to the same criteria that would be used in a neonate. Accurate estimation of fetal weight, however, is not easy. The large number of techniques that have been devised suggest that we have still not found a truly dependable method of measuring weight in utero, particularly when fetuses at either extreme of the weight spectrum are considered. Lind (19) has pointed out that by simply guessing that each fetus at term weighs 3.3 kg, one would be within 454 g of the true weight 70% of the time. This is a minimum standard against which to measure any technique for estimating fetal weight. Several publications in the 1960's suggested that predictions of fetal weight using BPD's alone were fairly inaccurate. This is not surprising for several reasons which have already been discussed. Investigators have studied other variables alone and in combination in an attempt to increase the precision with which fetal weight can be assessed in utero.

Abdominal circumference In 1975 Campbell and Wilkin (7) devised a nomogram for birth weight vs. fetal abdominal circumference based on measurements from 140 fetuses who delivered within 48 hrs. of the ultrasound examination (see Appendix). At a predicted weight of 1000 g, 95% of birth weights fell within 160 g, while at 2000, 3000, and 4000 g the corresponding values were 290, 450, and 590 g, respectively. The percentage of deviation from true birth weight, however, remained constant throughout this range. An important problem with this technique is that the splay within 95% confidence limits may be quite large. For example, an abdominal circumference of 36 cm corresponds to a weight of 3640 g at the 50th percentile, but ranges from 3180 to 4160 g at the 5th and 95th percentiles, respectively, a difference of almost 1000 g from one extreme to the other.

Higginbottom et al. (14) published their results using abdominal circumferences to predict birth weights in 50 cases. In 94% the birth weight was within 145 g of the predicted value with a maximum error of 225 g Kurjak and Breyer (17), using their own nomogram to estimate birth weights from fetal abdominal circumference, were within 250 g 94% of the time. The mean error was 105 g with a maximum error of 310 g. These authors, however, discarded a 620-g error from their series. Poll and Kasby (28) described a method where the abdominal circumference was converted into a weight percentile for gestational age and then weight predicted from birth weight data generated by Thomson et al. (31). Their mean error between actual and predicted weights was 194 g for all patients. When the BPD corresponded to a gestational age within 1 week of dates calculated from LMP, 22 of 25 patients were within 175 g. This paper, by the way, contains a table referencing 13 other studies of fetal weight estimations.

Kurjak et al. (18) have analyzed their ultrasound data on 260 pregnancies which resulted in SGA babies. Abdominal circumference measurement was found to be the most accurate single ultrasonic technique in identifying fetuses with IUGR. Abdominometry indicated that 84% of 62 SGA fetuses had values below the 10th percentile. This compares favorably to 49% of 72 single BPD's, 52% of 188 serial BPD studies, 59% of 70 HFUPR's, and 80% of 51 H:A ratios being below the 10th percentile in cases of IUGR. By combining their abdominal circumference measurements with single cephalometry, these authors were able to diagnose intrauterine growth retardation in 97% of cases.

Combinations of ultrasound measurements A number of papers have been published describing techniques for estimating fetal weight which utilize various combinations of ultrasonically derived measurements. These methods often require the use of complex mathematical equations to convert the data measured into estimated weights. They are all based, however, on the principle that fetal area or volume measurements correspond to weight. Mass is equal to volume times density. The precise density of fetal tissue may be altered somewhat as it matures because of the accumulation of more body fat, but Morrison and McLennan feel that this change is probably of minimal significance (26). The overall density of the fetus, when all the component tissues have been considered, is very close to 1.0. Therefore, it seems reasonable to pursue measurements of size in an attempt to predict weight in utero, but the accurate measurement of fetal volume remains an elusive goal.

Morrison and McLennan (26), using multiple parallel scans to derive fetal volume, had a standard error of 106 g in predicting birth weight in 20 patients. Issel and Prenzlau (16) used skull, thoracic, and longitudinal measurements to estimate weight in utero. These authors derived three different formulas for calculating EFW's. The first was for fetuses thought to be in the normal range, the second was for very small fetuses, and the third was "a good check method" for all fetuses. Lunt and Chard (22) used a combination of skull and thoracic area measurements. Picker and Saunders (27) advocated calculating the volume of the head and abdomen, conceptualized as a cylinder, by using the BPD and distance from the tip of the fetal head to the inferior aspect of the fetal bladder. To this they added the volume of the four limbs which was calculated after measuring the width of an upper thigh and the distance from hip to knee. McCallum and Brinkley (25) took serial scanning cuts through the sagittal and transverse axis of the fetus and subjected their data to multiple regression analyses. The formula giving the best correlation was a polynomial regression of the natural logarithm of birth weight vs. trunk circumference, circumference^2, and a specific long axis measurement referred to as "arch length." This method gave an approximate standard error of 103 g/kg.

Birnholz (2) has published a formula for estimating fetal weight using cranial biparietal and occipito-frontal diameters, along with average AP and transverse abdominal diameters. The constants for this formula were derived by regression analysis of 132 consecutive cases with ultrasound measurements within several hours of delivery. In a study population spanning 500 to 4000 g, the reported standard error with this technique was 112 g.

In 1977 we published a technique for estimating fetal weight based on measurements of the BPD and AC (34). The formula used was derived from multiple variable linear regressions of all possible combinations of BPD and AC measured against known birth weight. The predictive accuracy of this formula used in a small prospective study was 106 g./kg. Tables were generated from the formula which permitted the ultrasonographer simply to cross match measured BPD's and AC's in order to obtain an EFW.

Continued use of these tables gave us the impression that we were often underestimating fetal weight. Therefore, with data obtained from 73 patients who delivered within 2 days of being scanned, an earlier unpublished equation (E2) was compared with the one used to generate the original tables (E1). While most estimates from both equations were within 10% of the actual weight, there was a significant underestimation with E1 (30). The average differences between actual and predicted weights were -130.2 g. for E1 and -12.8 g. for E2. Twenty-six percent of the predictions from E2 were within 5% of the birth weight as compared to 23% from E1. Furthermore, the accuracy of E2 was maintained for each subset when the study population was divided into birth weights <2500 g, 2500 to 3500 g, and >3500 g. We, therefore, feel that E2 should be substituted for our previously published equation. The new formula and tables derived from it are presented in the Appendix.

Most of the methods described above for estimating weight in utero have comparable predictive values. Many of them, however, involve taking multiple measurements and/or making complicated calculations. We continue to advocate our own method because it is easy to perform, reproducible, and has proven its efficacy in hundreds of cases.

Ideally, we would like to be able to predict fetal weight with unerring accuracy. While this cannot be done now, it may become possible when newer technology permits us to rapidly perform serial scanning cuts separated by constant distances. The computerized integration of these scans would then produce accurate three-dimensional models from which precise volume measurements could be derived. The conversion from volume to weight should be fairly straightforward except in well-defined pathological conditions such as hydrops. Until the technical capacity to obtain measurements of this nature has developed, however, the techniques currently available provide very useful tools for approximating weight in utero.

Integrated approach to the diagnosis of IUGR

Our approach to the ultrasonic diagnosis of IUGR is outlined in Table 1. While the table is self-explanatory, a number of points should be stressed. A common and frequent problem in diagnosing IUGR is that the patient often has her initial scan performed in the third trimester following referral to rule out IUGR. If her dates are uncertain, the BPD is the only objective method of assessing gestational age at that time. In addition to the inherent difficulties of dating based on BPD after 30 weeks, an additional factor may be diminution of that variable by IUGR. If, on the other hand, the dates are "known" and they are discrepant with the BPD, there may be head involvement secondary to IUGR or, alternatively, the dates may be incorrect. For these reasons it is frequently necessary to perform serial scans in order to determine gestational age more accurately as well as to follow the progress of growth in utero. In other words, several examinations may be necessary in order to simply diagnose IUGR, not just to follow its course.

In our scheme TIUV is used as a screening test. If it is normal and compatible with dates, it is extremely unlikely that IUGR is present. If, on the other hand, it is abnormally low, further studies are needed. When real-time equipment is used for the initial examination, the TIUV may be impossible to measure because of limitations caused by the transducer head length. In these cases, the sonographer may substitute an

Table 1

BPD and TIUV	Diagnosis	Disposition
1. BPD ⎱ Both appropriate for dates TIUV ⎰	No IUGR	No follow-up necessary unless clinical parameters warrant it.
2. BPD ⎱ Both 3 to 4 weeks off TIUV ⎰	Incorrect dates	Repeat scan once in 2 to 3 weeks to check for appropriate growth of BPD and TIUV.
3. BPD—Appropriate for dates TIUV—Small for dates	r/o Early asymmetrical IUGR	Complete profile.* Repeat every 2 weeks until delivery Treat for IUGR.†
4. BPD—<3 or >5 weeks behind dates TIUV—Appropriate for the BPD measured	Incorrect dates vs. Symmetrical IUGR	Complete profile.* Repeat every 2 weeks × 3, if growth is abnormally slow; continue every 2 weeks until delivery. Treat for IUGR† until this diagnosis has been ruled out. If symmetrical IUGR is diagnosed, look for anomalies and consider amniocentesis for karyotype.
5. BPD—Small for dates TIUV—Small for the BPD measured	Significant IUGR	Complete profile*; look for anomalies. Repeat every 2 weeks until delivery. Treat for IUGR.†

* A complete profile consists of AC, H:A ratio, EFW, TIUV, and placental grading.
† Treatment for IUGR consists of weekly electronic fetal heart rate monitoring, bed rest on the left side, cessation or decrease in smoking, increase in protein content of diet, and correction of anemia.

evaluation of amniotic fluid volume for a measured TIUV. This may be done either by rendering a subjective impression of the amount of fluid present or by using the minimal criterion of a pocket of fluid measuring at least 1 cm in its largest dimension. If either of these approaches is used, however, we would urge the sonographer to err on the side of overestimating oligohydramnios. It is better to perform a full profile and find it to be normal than to miss a case of IUGR.

A complete scanning profile consists of BPD, TIUV, abdominal and head circumferences, and placental grading. Calculations are then made for H:A ratios and EFW. If the diagnosis of IUGR is seriously entertained, all of these parameters should be studied in a serial fashion in order to follow the progress of growth in utero. Once diagnosed, an IUGR fetus should have non-stress test and, if necessary, contraction stress tests performed at least once a week until the time of delivery.

In cases of suspected symmetrical IUGR, an attempt should be made to rule out congenital anomalies. Amniocentesis should be considered for chromosomal analysis if the quantity of amniotic fluid is relatively

Figure 8

Sagittal scan of a pregnancy with severe oligohydramnios at term. This fetus had renal agenesis.

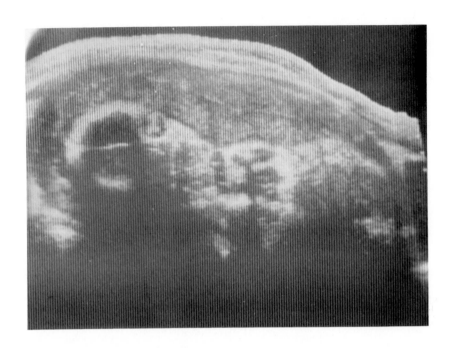

normal for the size of the fetus. Historical inquiry should be made into viral, radiation or teratogenic exposure during the first trimester. Finally, when severe oligohydramnios is present, the fetal kidneys and bladder should be examined to rule out significant renal dysfunction (Figure 8).

Management of IUGR

Beischer and Brown (1) reported increased estriol excretion into the normal range in 27% of 184 patients with subnormal values who were treated with bed rest in the lateral position. We have also seen ultrasonic evidence of a dramatic increase in fetal growth when women were admitted to the hospital and put to bed. This, of course, makes sense since bed rest reduces the requirements of peripheral muscles and consequently increases the amount of oxygenated blood available for flow to the uterus. Furthermore, lying on the side removes uterine pressure on both the aorta and vena cava and maximizes the potential for effective cardiovascular performance. This form of therapy is, therefore, quite rational, and in some patients it is capable of producing dramatic results. In addition to bed rest other useful therapeutic maneuvers include elimination, or at least reduction, of cigarette smoking, correction of significant anemia, and dietary augmentation with increased protein.

While these approaches are fairly straightforward, there are two important areas in which controversy exists. The first of these is in regard to the management of a woman with IUGR secondary to hypertension. Assuming that there are no maternal or fetal indications for immediate delivery, at what level should the maternal blood pressure be maintained while the measures mentioned above are being tried? Is it better to use vasodilator therapy to lower diastolic pressure to around 90 mmHg in an attempt to open up constricted uterine vasculature, or should this value be kept closer to 110 mmHg in women with normal eye grounds in order to maintain high perfusion pressures to the placental bed? We know that under normal circumstances the uterine arteries are maximally dilated, but is this true in the woman with hypertension in pregnancy? Is the effect gained by opening up a constricted utero-placental circulation lost by decreasing systemic pressure? The answers to these questions are not agreed upon. Our approach is to try to maintain maternal diastolic pressures between 100 and 110 mm.Hg. as we have seen electronic fetal heart rate monitoring (EFM) evidence of fetal distress in hypersensitive women whose blood pressures have rapidly dropped into the normal range. Obviously, however, more work must be done in this complicated area, as it is possible that some fetuses might benefit from a reduction in maternal blood pressure to values lower than those we seek to achieve.

A second important area of controversy is the management of a pregnancy prior to 37 weeks when a fetus is growth-retarded and has a mature L/S ratio (15). Some clinicians feel that unless there is EFM evidence of fetal distress, these patients should not be delivered until 37 or 38 weeks. This approach avoids the potential increase in cesarean sections associated with inductions in women with unripe cervices. It also avoids the many problems other than RDS which may affect premature neonates. However, other physicians feel that once pulmonic maturity has been obtained, it is worth these risks to remove a fetus from suboptimal surroundings into those where its respiratory and nutritive needs can be maximally met. We subscribe to the latter viewpoint. We are concerned about the possibility that ongoing chronic nutritional deprivation in utero may have long lasting subtle developmental effects. The premature infant who does not suffer hypoxic brain insult in utero or in the nursery has, by and large, been shown to have an excellent long term prognosis. We, therefore, favor the delivery of growth-retarded babies as soon as pulmonic maturity has been documented. We recognize that the validity of either of the two approaches mentioned has not been convincingly demonstrated to date and hope that well-controlled studies will be performed to provide us with meaningful data on this issue. It must be recognized, however, that large numbers of neonates will have to be studied and the developmental follow-up should be carried out for at least 5 to 10 years.

If no amniotic fluid is obtainable to study indices of pulmonic maturity, we hospitalize the patients and follow the infant with non-stress tests and/or contraction stress tests twice a week. If after 33 weeks there has been no ultrasonically demonstrable fetal growth in a 2-week interval and a grade 3 placenta is evident, we advocate delivery even in the absence of fetal distress on EFM.

Conclusions

Intrauterine growth retardation is a common and potentially devastating problem. With the intelligent use of ultrasound, EFM, and amniocentesis the morbidity and mortality associated with this condition can be significantly reduced.

References

1 **Beischer, N.A., Brown, J.B.:** Current status of estrogen assays in obstetrics and gynecology. Obstet. Gynecol. Surv. 27:303, 1972.

2 **Birnholz, J.C.:** Ultrasound characterization of fetal growth. Ultrasonic Imaging 2:135, 1980.

3 **Butler, N.R., Alberman, E.D.:** *Perinatal Problems: The Second Report of the British Perinatal Mortality Survey.* Churchill Livingstone, Edinburgh, 1969.

4 **Campbell, S.:** Physical methods of assessing size at birth. In *Size at Birth.* CIBA Foundation Symposium 27, Associated Scientific Publishers, Amsterdam, 1974, p. 275.

5 **Campbell, S., Dewhurst, C. J.:** Diagnosis of the small-for-dates fetus by serial ultrasonic cephalometry. Lancet 2:1002, 1971.

6 **Campbell, S., Thoms, A.:** Ultrasound measurement of the fetal head-to-abdomen circumference ratio in the assessment of growth retardation. Br. J. Obstet. Gynaecol. 84:165, 1977.

7 **Campbell, S., Wilkin, D.:** Ultrasonic measurement of fetal abdomen circumference in the estimation of fetal weight. Br. J. Obstet. Gynaecol. 82:689, 1975.

8 **Campbell, S., Wladimiroff, J.W., Dewhurst, C.J.:** The antenatal measurement of fetal urine production. J. Obstet. Gynaecol. Br. Commonw. 80:680, 1973.

9 **Clement, D., Silverman, R., Scott, D., Hobbins, J.C.:**
Comparison of abdominal circumference measurements by
real-time and B-scan techniques. J. Clin. Ultrasound 9:1, 1981.

10 **DeVore, G.R., Hobbins, J.C.:** Fetal growth and development:
The diagnosis of intrauterine growth retardation. Clin. Diagn.
Ultrasound 3:81, 1979.

11 **Fancourt, R., Campbell, S., Harvey, D., Norman, A.P.:**
Follow-up study of small-for-dates babies. Br. Med. J. 1:1435,
1976.

12 **Fitzhardinge, P.M., Steven, E.M.:** The small-for-date infant. II.
Neurological and intellectual sequelae. J. Pediatr. 49:50, 1972.

13 **Gohari, P., Berkowitz, R.L., Hobbins, J.C.:** Prediction of
intrauterine growth retardation by determination of total
intrauterine volume. Am. J. Obstet. Gynecol. 127:255, 1977.

14 **Higginbottom, J., Slater, J., Porter, G., Whitfield, C. R.:**
Estimation of fetal weight from ultrasonic measurement of trunk
circumference. Br. J. Obstet. Gynaecol. 82:698, 1975.

15 **Hobbins, J.C., Berkowitz, R.L., Grannum, P.A.T.:** Diagnosis
and antepartum management of intrauterine growth retardation.
J. Repro. Med. 21:319, 1978.

16 **Issel, E.P., Prenzlau, F.L.:** Problems in using linear ultrasound
parameters for the determination of fetal weight. J. Perinat. Med.
4:26, 1976.

17 **Kurjak, A., Breyer, B.:** Estimation of fetal weight by ultrasonic
abdominometry. Am. J. Obstet. Gynecol. 125:962, 1976.

18 **Kurjak, A., Kirkinen, P., Latin, V.:** Biometric and dynamic
ultrasound assessment of small-for-dates infants: Report of 260
cases. Obstet. Gynecol. 56:281, 1980.

19 **Lind, T.:** The estimation of fetal growth and development. Br. J.
Hosp. Med. 3:501, 1970.

20 **Loeffler, F.E.:** Clinical foetal weight prediction. J. Obstet.
Gynaecol. Br. Commonw. 74:675, 1967.

21 **Low, J.A., Galbraith, R.L.:** Pregnancy characteristics of
intrauterine growth retardation. Obstet. Gynecol. 44:122, 1974.

22 **Lunt, R., Chard, T.:** A new method for estimation of fetal weight
in late pregnancy by ultrasonic scanning. Br. J. Obstet.
Gynaecol. 83:1, 1976.

23 **Manning, F.A., Hill, L.M., Platt, L.D.:** Qualitative amniotic fluid
volume determination by ultrasound: Antepartum detection of
intrauterine growth retardation. Am. J. Obstet. Gynecol.
139:254, 1981.

24 **Martinez, D.A., Barton, J.L.:** Estimation of fetal body and fetal
head volumes: Description of technique and nomograms for 18
to 41 weeks of gestation. Am. J. Obstet. Gynecol. 137:78,
1980.

25 **McCallum, W.D., Brinkley, J.F.:** Estimation of fetal weight from
ultrasonic measurements. Am. J. Obstet. Gynecol. 133:195,
1979.

26   **Morrison, J., McLennan, M.J.:** The theory, feasibility and accuracy of an ultrasonic method of estimating fetal weight. Br. J. Obstet. Gynaecol. 83:833, 1976.

27   **Picker, R. H., Saunders, D.M.:** A simple geometric method for determining fetal weight in utero with the compound gray scale ultrasonic scan. Am. J. Obstet. Gynecol. 124:493, 1976.

28   **Poll, V., Kasby, C.B.:** An improved 'method of fetal weight estimation using ultrasound measurements of fetal abdominal circumference. Br. J. Obstet. Gynaecol. 86:922, 1979.

29   **Sabbagha, R.E.:** Intrauterine growth retardation: Antenatal diagnosis by ultrasound. Obstet. Gynecol. 52:252, 1978.

30   **Shepard, M.J., Richards, V.A., Berkowitz, R.L., Warsof, S.L., Hobbins, J.C.:** An evaluation of two equations for predicting fetal weight by ultrasound. Am. J. Obstet. Gynecol. 142:47, 1982.

31   **Thomson, A.M., Billewicz, W.Z., Hytten, F.E.:** The assessment of fetal growth. J. Obstet. Gynaecol Br. Commonw. 75:903, 1968.

32   **Usher, R.H., McLean, F.H.:** Normal fetal growth and the significance of fetal growth retardation. In *Scientific Foundations of Paediatrics*, J.A. Davis, J. Dobbing, eds. Heineman, London, 1974, p. 69.

33   **Warshaw, J.B.:** The growth retarded fetus. Clin. Perinatol. 6:353, 1979.

34   **Warsof, S.L., Gohari, P., Berkowitz, R.L., Hobbins, J.C.:** The estimation of fetal weight by computer-assisted analysis. Am. J. Obstet. Gynecol. 128:881, 1977.

35   **Weiner, C.P., Sabbagha, R.E., Tamura, R.K., DalCompo, S.:** Sonographic abdominal circumference: Dynamic versus static imaging. Am. J. Obstet. Gynecol. 139:953, 1981.

36   **Wilcox, A.J.:** Birth weight, gestation, and the fetal growth curve. Am. J. Obstet. Gynecol. 139:863, 1981.

37   **Winick, M., Brasel, J.A., Velasco, E.G.:** Effects of prenatal nutrition upon pregnancy risk. Clin. Obstet. Gynecol. 16:184, 1973.

38   **Wladimiroff, J.W., Bloemsma, C.A., Wallenburg, H.C.S.:** Ultrasonic assessment of fetal head and body sizes in relation to normal and retarded fetal growth. Am. J. Obstet. Gynecol. 131:857, 1978.

39   **Wladimiroff, J.W., Campbell, S.:** Fetal urine production rates in normal and complicated pregnancy. Lancet 1:151, 1974.

Normal and Abnormal Fetal Anatomy

7

Prenatal diagnosis of congenital anomalies is one of the major objects of and indications for ultrasonic examination. In many cases patients at increased risk of delivering an infant with an anomaly are now being examined by operators with considerable experience in the antenatal diagnosis of birth defects. However, very few anomalous infants are heralded by history or clinical clues; therefore, every examination, regardless of its initial indication, should include a rapid but systematic search for fetal abnormalities. The quality of modern double-focused linear arrays and mechanical sector scanners is such that the examination is first carried out with real-time equipment since rapidity and flexibility are achieved without significant loss of resolution. The articulated static scanner is sometimes necessary to supplement the linear array because of the limited access and lateral resolution of the latter. However, adequate transverse sections of spheroid structures such as the fetal spine and kidney can be obtained with a high quality real-time sector scanner, and such scans are easier to produce than with a static articulated scanner.

The examination should begin with a survey of the orientation of the fetus (or fetuses), placenta, and amniotic fluid. Amniotic fluid contains particulate matter that is visible with high resolution dynamic scanners as early as the 16th week (Figure 1). These reflectors move with fetal motion or operator pressure. Either increased or diminished amniotic fluid volume may be the first indicator of fetal anomalies. About 2% of patients have ultrasonically detectable excessive amniotic fluid, and about 18% of these women have an anomalous fetus (19) (Figure 2). In many cases polyhydramnios is secondary to impairment of fetal swallowing, but in some syndromes the mechanisms by which excessive amounts of fluid accumulate are unknown. Polyhydramnios may be associated with abnormalities of the central nervous system, gastrointestinal system, and a few skeletal dysplasias. It should be suspected when TIUV is 1 S.D. above the mean for gestation and is diagnosed by the

Figure 1
Midterm pregnancy with particulate matter evident in amniotic fluid.

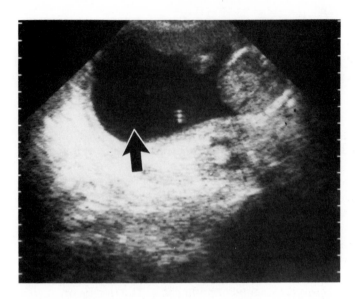

identification of large amounts of fluid separating the fetal small parts.

If there is oligohydramnios in the second trimester, a fetal anomaly involving the urinary tract should be strongly suspected, but after the 28th week of gestation obstetrical complications such as premature rupture of membranes, asymmetrical IUGR, or post-term pregnancies may be responsible for the decreased amniotic fluid.

Cranium
Normal anatomy

Although examination of the fetal head has been performed for many years to measure the BPD, accurate measurement requires the recognition of anatomical landmarks that could not be appreciated with older real-time equipment and were too difficult to locate consistently with static scanners. Sections through the base of the skull show the X-shaped sphenoid wings and temporal bones (Figure 3). The midbrain and cerebral peduncles are the easiest landmarks to identify. These have a heart-shaped form with the apex pointing posteriorly. The basilar artery can be seen pulsating in the midline at the base of the "heart" (peduncles), and the posterior cerebral arteries course around the midbrain in the paramesencephalic cisterns. The aqueduct lies in the midbrain and is occasionally seen as a bright reflection (Figure 4a and b).

Figure 2

Transverse scan showing polyhydramnios.

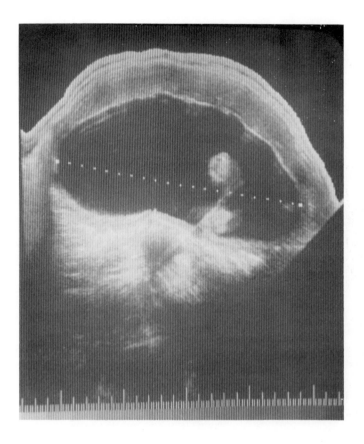

Behind the peduncles either the falx or cerebellum is imaged depending on the obliquity of the section. Just above the midbrain plane but below the ventricular plane one can locate the rounded thalami, and the third ventricle is sometimes visible between the thalami. Other structures often seen in the thalamic plane include the frontal horns, the cavum septi pellucidi (22), the medial aspect of the temporal lobe (probably the hippocampal gyrus), and the temporal horns of the lateral ventricle or the Sylvian fissures (Figure 5). (Since the angle of section with respect to the baseline varies slightly, there are minor variations to all these patterns, but this level is considered the best for measurement of the BPD.) The ventricular plane lies superior to the thalamic plane and is the next to be examined. It shows the bodies of the lateral ventricles. (Figure 6).

The lateral ventricles are largely filled with strongly echogenic choroid plexuses in the first 18 weeks of the

Figure 3

Axial section through base of skull. *Arrows* point to temporal bones (petrous pyramids). *A*, anterior fossa; *P*, posterior fossa; *M*, middle fossa; *O*, occiput.

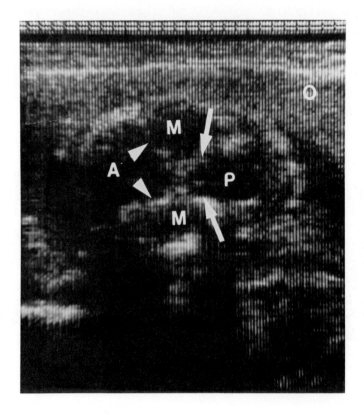

pregnancy (Figure 7). (The choroid may be a source of glycogen for the developing cerebrum.) The frontal horns are relatively easy to identify and measure, serving as an indicator of ventricular size. The bifrontal diameter (distance from the lateral margin of one frontal horn to the lateral margin of the opposite frontal horn) is about 50% of the biparietal diameter at 15 weeks, diminishing to about 25% at term. Most articles in the literature compare the width of one ventricle to the diameter of the cerebral hemisphere at the level of the measurement, that is, from the midline to the inner table of the skull. Although this is a logical "ventricular ratio," we believe it is simpler to divide the biventricular diameter by the BPD. If one uses the frontal horn/cerebral hemisphere ratio, the values are higher, ranging from 80% at 15 weeks to about 35% at term (Figure 8).

One should not confuse the Sylvian fissures or temporal horns with the lateral walls of the lateral

Figure 4

Axial sections through midbrain. *a. Arrows* point to temporal horns of
lateral ventricles. *S*, aqueduct of Sylvius. *b. Arrows* point to cerebral
peduncles. Bright echo (*large arrow*) represents basilar artery.

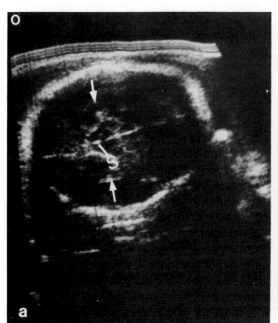
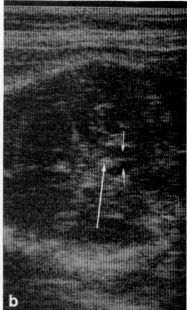

ventricles. They are located in the plane of the thalami
and are consequently at a more caudal level than the
lateral walls of the lateral ventricles. The Sylvian
fissures can be identified by their curvature and the
pulsations of the middle cerebral arteries (Figure 9).

It is interesting to observe the fetal face between 16 to
20 weeks, although anomalies are rarely identified
(Figure 10). The orbits are easy to visualize, and the
lenses are echogenic structures occupying the anterior
portion of the orbits (Figure 11). During short periods of
observation one sometimes observes ocular
movements whose character may be associated with
neurological development of the fetus. This is currently
a research concept and is under investigation.
Measurements of the extra- and intraorbital distances
correlate extremely well with the BPD (28), and when
the fetus is in a face-up position the extraorbital
diameter can be used in lieu of the unmeasurable BPD
for estimation of gestational age (see Appendix). Also,
these measurements are useful in conditions in which
hypo- or hypertelorism is a feature, such as
holoprosencephaly, fetal alcohol syndrome, or Apert
syndrome.

Figure 5

Axial section of the head through the level of the thalami. (*T*), *SF*, Sylvian fissure.

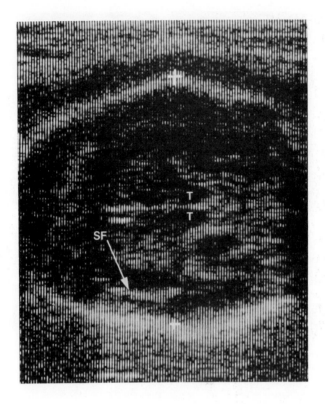

Observation of the mandible shows yawning and swallowing as well as thumb sucking and face scratching. Dental buds can be observed as early as 16 weeks and isolated instances of cleft palate have been diagnosed.

Hydrocephaly

Congenitally acquired hydrocephaly (without other neural tube defects) occurs in 1:2000 live births. The recurrence rate of communicating hydrocephaly is less than 4%, but aqueductal stenosis is sometimes inherited as an X-linked recessive trait with a 50% recurrence rate in male fetuses (Figure 12), and obstruction of the foramina of Luschka and Magendie (Dandy-Walker syndrome) is inherited as an autosomal recessive trait with a 25% recurrence rate (21). About 80% of affected newborns not diagnosed in utero are diagnosed by the first year of age (36).

With hydrocephalus due to obstruction of the aqueduct or 4th ventricle or secondary to spina bifida (Arnold-Chiari malformation), high pressures build up inside the ventricles even before the skull enlarges to abnormal

Figure 6

Axial section through bodies of lateral ventricles (*LV*).

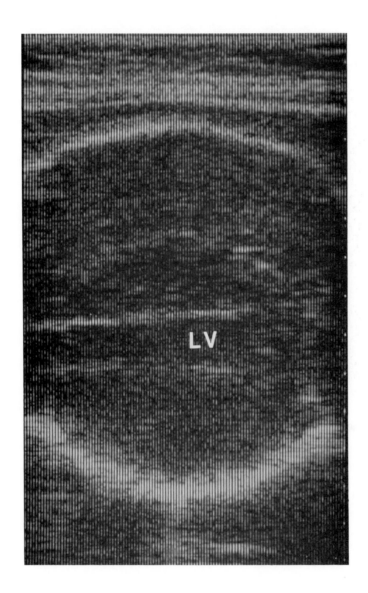

proportions. For example, during a procedure to shunt obstructed cerebrospinal fluid into the amniotic cavity through a catheter at 27 weeks we measured the interventricular pressure to be 35 cm water. Elevated pressure results in myelin destruction and compression of the cerebral mantle.

Since increased intraventricular pressure precedes ventricular dilatation and studies of neonatal

Figure 7

Axial section through bodies of the lateral ventricles (*V*) at 19 weeks of gestation. *c*, choroid plexi.

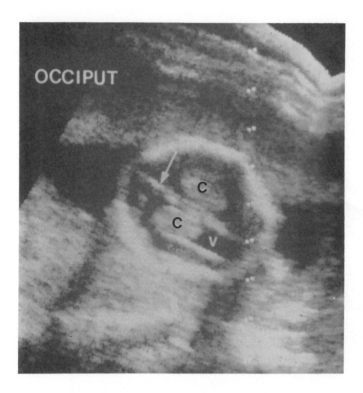

hydrocephalus have shown that vertical and medial dilatation of the ventricles precedes lateral dilatation, increase in the ventricular ratio does not occur until hydrocephalus is well advanced. Even then, enlargement of the occipital horns seems to precede enlargement of the frontal horns. Despite these potential limitations to the use of ventricular size as an indicator of hydrocephalus, the intrauterine diagnosis of hydrocephalus is rarely a difficult problem. Although there are probably cases in which hydrocephalus develops late in pregnancy, it is our impression that lateral ventricular dilatation is generally present before the 24th week. Without doubt, ventricular dilatation precedes enlargement of the skull (Figure 13). In cases of hydrocephaly that have been followed serially, it is rare for the BPD to be abnormally enlarged until the 28th week of gestation. At term, however, the BPD can be as much as 12 cm. (Figure 14). As knowledge about intracranial anatomy is disseminated and ultrasound instruments improve, one can anticipate that better early signs of hydrocephalus will be described. However, since no one would attempt to treat an ''early'' intrauterine hydrocephalus surgically and

Figure 8

Coronal section through fetal head near term showing frontal horns (*arrows*). Below the frontal horns lie the thalami (*t*).

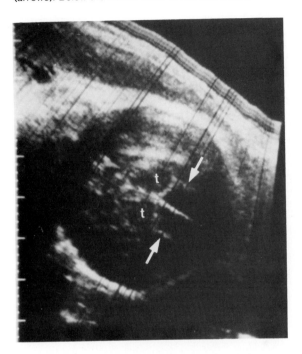

abortion is not justified, the clinical usefulness of this knowledge is problematic.

Anencephaly

Anencephaly is a defect of cranial development involving the frontal, parietal, and occipital bones with subsequent necrosis of the developing cerebral hemispheres. The etiology appears to be multifactorial, with both genetic and environmental components that affect the embryo between the 16th and 26th postconceptual day. The incidence varies from as high as 1:105 births in South Wales to 1:1000 births in other parts of the world (35). All fetuses die either in utero or shortly after birth.

The diagnosis of anencephaly is readily made in the second trimester. In the past these patients were referred because the uterus was large-for-dates due to hydramnios secondary to abnormal swallowing by an affected fetus, but more recently the diagnosis is usually an incidental finding during a screening examination. The fetal body is easily identified, fetal movements may be vigorous, and the fetal heart is readily located, but only a primordial fetal head that includes facial bones and prominent orbits is attached

Figure 9

Axial section through the thalami showing Sylvian fissure (*SF*); *ML*, midline echoes; *CP*, cerebral peduncles.

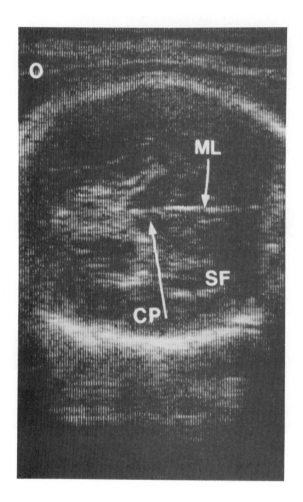

to the fetal body (Figure 15). Occasionally, on cursory ultrasound examination, a normal fetal head cannot be identified when the cranium is deep in the pelvis. Before concluding that the fetus is anencephalic, a pelvic examination should be performed to lift the head out of the pelvis. Radiography is confirmatory in the third trimester.

Microcephaly

Microcephaly can result from many causes such as chromosome disorders, fetal alcohol syndrome, or TORCH infections. Little information is available concerning how early in gestation the BPD falls below the normal curve, but in four cases we have studied two fetuses had abnormal BPD's before the 24th week of gestation and two did not. Since a small BPD might simply represent a fetus whose dates were in error,

Figure 10
Fetal face in profile.

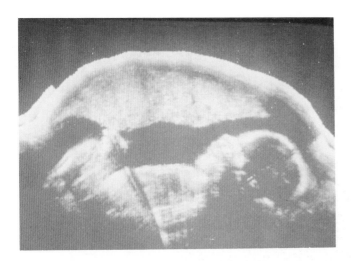

comparison with other body measurements, such as the femoral length or abdominal circumference, is necessary. In microcephaly the head-to-body ratio eventually falls to the 5th percentile, but early in pregnancy this ratio may be normal.

Encephalocele

Encephalocele occurs in 1:2000 live births. In these infants a defect is present in the calvarium through which brain tissue protrudes. Encephalocele may occur in combination with microcephaly and polycystic kidneys (Meckel syndrome) (32). Encephalocele with or without other abnormalities is a condition with very poor prognosis but, fortunately, a very low recurrence rate (Figure 16).

Cystic hygroma

The ultrasound appearance of cystic hygromas is classic (11, 19). They are multiloculated cystic structures on either side of the fetal neck and head and may be larger than the fetal head (Figure 17). Since cystic hygromas most often are associated with Turner syndrome, we advocate obtaining amniotic fluid for karyotyping whenever they are diagnosed. The spectrum of findings with this condition can range from associated hydrops with severe edema and ascites to isolated nuchal cysts. One investigator has observed

Figure 11

Transverse scan through a fetal skull showing the orbits. The inner and outer margins of each orbit are marked with *crosses*. *ML*, midline echoes.

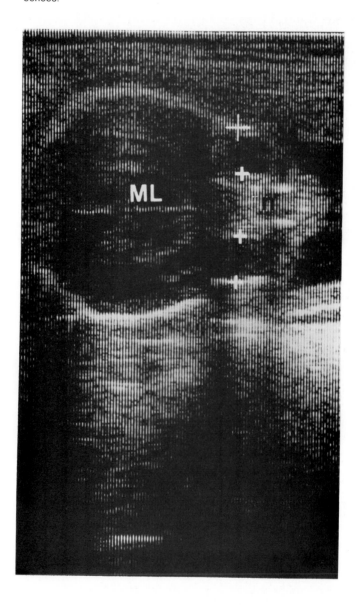

regression of small cystic hygromas as pregnancy progressed. The fetus was born with a webbed neck but without the cystic hygromas observed in the first scan. This observation could explain the etiology of the nuchal webbing in Turner syndrome. Nevertheless, Turner syndrome is a lethal condition for many fetuses, and the chances of a fetus surviving once huge cystic hygromas and the stigmata of non-immune hydrops are seen is probably remote. One should not mistake a cystic hygroma for a cervical or cranial meningocele.

Figure 12

Aqueductal stenosis showing dilated lateral ventricle (*LV*) and dilated third ventricle (*arrow*).

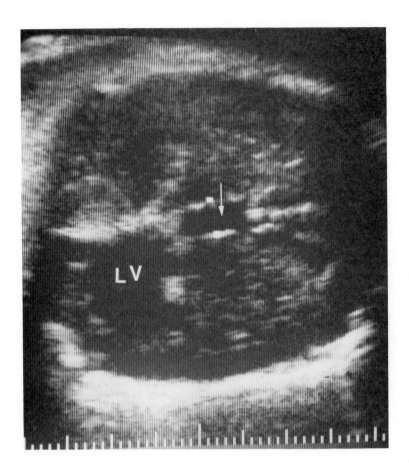

Spine

Spina bifida can be divided into two major groups, spina bifida occulta and spina bifida cystica. Spina bifida occulta is associated with a number of other congenital malformation syndromes, but in itself rarely leads to any neurological deficit. Spina bifida cystica (myelomeningocele), however, is associated with neurological deficit in more than 90% of cases, and it occurs with a frequency varying between 1:200 to 1:500 live births in the British Isles and about 1:1000 live births in North America (4). The genetics are multifactorial, with a recurrence rate from 3% to 7% for a fetus with a previously affected sibling or a fetus of an affected parent.

Fifty percent of fetuses born alive survive longer than 5 years and of these 25% are mentally retarded (36).

Figure 13

Hydrocephaly at 20 weeks in a fetus with a normal BPD. *White arrow* points to lateral border of lateral ventricle. *Black arrow* points to choroid plexus.

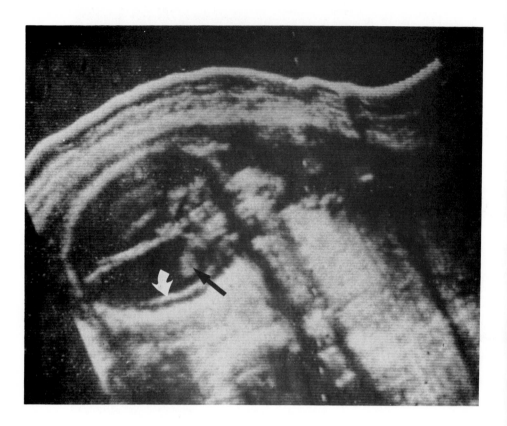

Although approximately 70% develop secondary hydrocephaly (Arnold-Chiari syndrome) (36), in our experience only about 40% show sonographic evidence of ventricular dilatation in the second or third trimesters. Spinal defects result from incomplete closure of the neural tube. If the defect is not covered with a full skin thickness, alphafetoprotein (AFP) leaks through the fetal meninges into the amniotic fluid (3) producing levels that are generally more than 5 standard deviations above the mean and resulting in elevated maternal serum AFP (MSAFP) levels. Measurement of the latter has been used as a screening method for the detection of neural tube defects. This is a sensitive method but of low specificity. For every 1000 second trimester patients screened with MSAFP, 50 to 70 have elevated levels (defined in most laboratories as above 2.5 multiples of the median or the equivalent of the 5th percentile). Ultrasound (stage I) then plays an invaluable role in

Figure 14

Hydrocephaly at term with an enlarged BPD (markers indicate margins of midline and lateral ventricle); the cerebral mantle measured <1 cm.

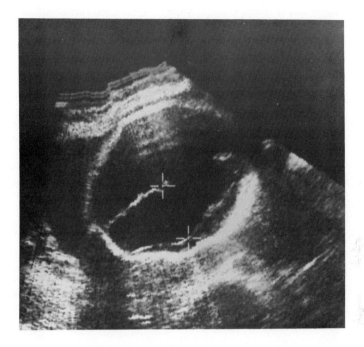

excluding those patients in the group with an elevated MSAFP who have a dead baby, twins, or erroneous dates. All of these situations are responsible for falsely high levels of MSAFP. Usually, about 20 patients of the original 1000 women will require further evaluation by amniocentesis after the above "stage I" ultrasound evaluation and one to two will have amniotic fluid AFP (AFAFP) levels greater than 5 S.D. above the mean. Another two to three will have elevations between 3 and 5 S.D. above the mean. According to earlier studies, the former group ran over a 90% risk (40) of having a neural tube defect, and the latter group was at risk for AFP-related abnormalities other than neural tube defects, such as ventral wall defects, upper gastrointestinal obstruction, cystic hygromas, later stillbirth, or premature labor.

We strongly suggest that a "stage II" examination be performed by individuals with considerable experience in detection of neural tube defects (NTD) before a decision is made to terminate pregnancy in those patients with high AFAFP's. A preliminary study from Yale-New Haven Hospital (20) suggests that an AFAFP

Figure 15

Second trimester anencephalic showing absence of cranium.

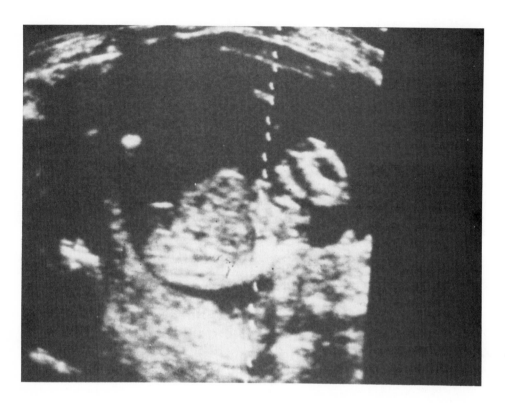

more than 5 S.D. above the mean is not definitely diagnostic of a neurologically significant NTD. Of 16 patients in this study with AFAFP levels 5 S.D. above the mean, six fetuses had spina bifida (one of which was very low and surgically correctable), four fetuses had ventral wall defects (three of which were potentially correctable), four fetuses were completely normal, one fetus had multiple lethal anomalies, and one fetus died later of unknown causes. The point that must be stressed here is that even very high AFAFP levels may be associated with perfectly normal fetuses. Only an expert ultrasound examination can distinguish those fetuses from their affected counterparts and avoid termination of normal pregnancy.

An isozyme of acetylcholinesterase has recently been used in conjunction with AFP to diagnose NTD's (38). The presence of acetyl cholinesterase in amniotic fluid is much more specific than AFP in predicting neural tube defects, and, therefore, it is particularly useful when combined with stage II ultrasound examinations once amniotic fluid AFP is elevated. At the present time

Figure 16

Encephalocele (*arrow*) in a fetus associated with hydrocephaly.

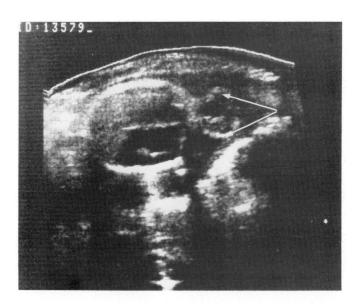

the analysis is more difficult than AFP, so it has not been used as a first line screening test.

In order to study the spine for defects, it is useful to understand the normal anatomy. In the second trimester the vertebral bodies contain three calcified ossification centers, the two posterolateral laminae and the anterior mass. Longitudinal sections through the laminae give the appearance of parallel lines with slight normal cervical widening and gradual sacral tapering (Figures 18 to 20). By rocking the real-time head in the plane of the spine, one can see the two lateral laminae and the midline alternately (Figure 21). With the best real-time equipment, the vertebral bodies can be individually identified as early as 14 weeks. With spina bifida there is either gross irregularity in the parallelism of the lines produced by the laminae or there is splaying or widening (Figure 22). Sections at right angle to the long axis of the spine show a rounded section in normal cases without divergence of the posterolateral elements (laminae) (Figure 23). With spina bifida the laminae diverge from the anterior mass and produce a cup or wedge-shaped pattern (Figure 24). Theoretically one should be able to detect divergence of the laminae by longitudinal sections alone, but it is generally considered good practice to study the spine completely with transverse sections,

Figure 17a

Transverse scan of a cystic hygroma posterior to the fetal head at 22
weeks. Notice the septum dividing large fluid-filled sac.

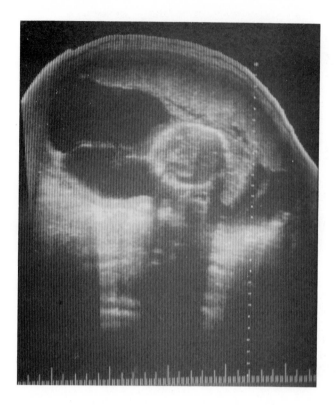

particularly to demonstrate soft tissue masses
protruding posteriorly. Transverse sections of the spine
are not adequately produced with a linear array and
require sectoring either manually or with real-time. It
should also be kept in mind that other anomalies, such
as hemivertebra, may result in irregularity of the spine
seen in long axis sections.

The visibility of meningoceles and meningomyeloceles
depends upon their being surrounded by amniotic fluid
and protuberant from the fetal back (Figure 25). If the
uterus is crowded and the sacculation lies against the
uterine wall or if there is oligohydramnios, these lesions
may be difficult to identify. Lesions without protruding
neural tissue can be missed on amniogram, and we,
therefore, do not recommend performing this
radiographic procedure for the diagnosis of NTD's.

Thorax

The fetal thorax may have an abnormal configuration in
certain skeletal dysplasias, such as thanatophoric
dwarfism, asphyxiating thoracic dystrophy, and

Figure 17b

Transverse scan through the abdomen of the same fetus. Notice the tremendous edema of the abdominal wall and the presence of ascites.

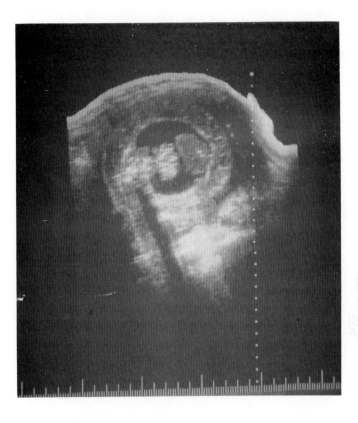

chondroectodermal dysplasia. In all of these situations the chest is quite narrow. Rib fractures have been detected in severe cases of osteogenesis imperfecta. The thorax is also hypoplastic in renal dysplasias, presumably because there is an insufficient quantity of amniotic fluid to expand the lungs. The association between oligohydramnios and pulmonary hypoplasia has been rather consistent; therefore, the hypothesis that hypoplasia results from curtailed lung expansion is widely accepted. The fact that ligation of the phrenic nerve in the fetal lamb results in hypoplastic lungs lends further credence to this theory. Yet oligohydramnios secondary to premature rupture of the

Figure 18

Parallel vertebral laminae in a fetus at 17 weeks.

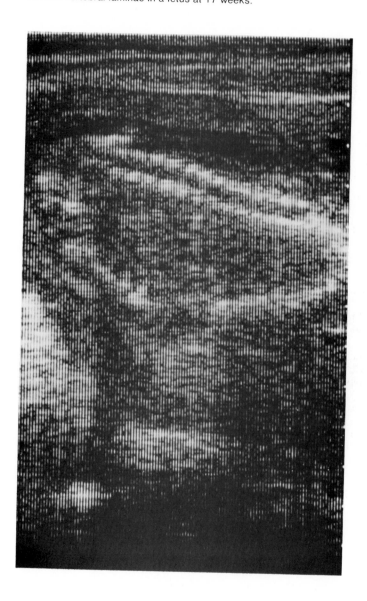

membranes (either spontaneous or secondary to fetoscopy) in the second trimester does not necessarily result in pulmonary hypoplasia, nor did breathing motions in five fetuses we observed with urinary tract anomalies seem to protect the fetuses against pulmonary hypoplasia. One must conclude, therefore, that the cause of pulmonary hypoplasia is not completely understood.

The fetal lungs are homogeneous low level reflectors delineated by a relatively transonic sliver at the level of the diaphragm (Figure 26). The diaphragm is best seen

Figure 19

Normal widening of the cervical spine at the base of the skull at 16 weeks.

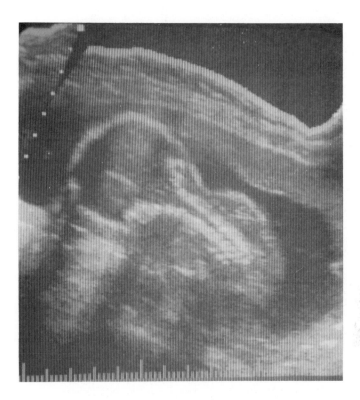

during respiratory excursions or below the heart, particularly at the entrance of the vena cava into the right atrium. With increasing maturity the reflectivity of the fetal lung approaches that of the liver, and it has been proposed that when echogenicity of the lung is equal to or greater than that of the liver pulmonary maturity has been achieved. Unfortunately, the lung is often seen through the acoustic window of the heart, and artifact may play a role in this judgment. Pleural effusions are readily visible between the lungs and diaphragm, and several rare anomalies have been observed, including congenital pulmonary tumors and thoracic cysts (Figure 27). If there is a large diaphragmatic hernia permitting the entrance of fluid-filled viscera into the thoracic cavity, it has the appearance of a fluid-filled mass in the thorax (19) (Figures 28a and 28b).

Diaphragmatic hernias can be classified anatomically as either the rare retrosternal defect which is usually not associated with neonatal pulmonary compromise or the posterolateral diaphragmatic defect which occurs in

Figure 20

Fetus showing narrowing of the sacral spine. *Large arrow* points to the sacrum and *small arrows* to the iliac wings.

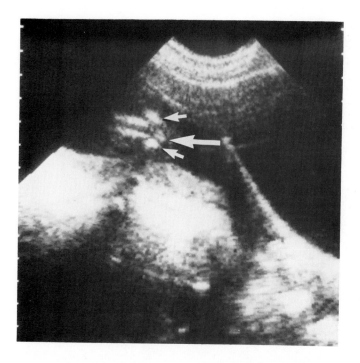

1:2200 live births. The posterolateral diaphragmatic hernia involves the left side of the diaphragm nine times more frequently than the right and is secondary to an insult that inhibits or delays normal migration of the gut and closure of the diaphragm between the 8th and 12th weeks of embryogenesis. Ninety percent of stillborn fetuses and 20% of liveborn infants with diaphragmatic hernias have other major anomalies that involve the central nervous, cardiovascular, genitourinary, and gastrointestinal systems (7).

Unfortunately, most newborns with posterolateral defects are not diagnosed prior to birth. Only after the baby develops cyanosis, dyspnea, pneumothorax, pneumomediastinum, hypoxia, acidosis, or even dies is the diagnosis suspected. Due to the delay in diagnosis, there is increased postnatal morbidity and mortality. If the defect is diagnosed prior to birth, appropriate neonatal preoperative preparation and rapid surgical repair can be performed with minimal risk.

Heart

With high resolution real-time scanners the cardiac chambers and valves can usually be well visualized. The four-chamber view showing the two ventricles, the

Figure 21

Spine of a normal 16-week fetus. *Vertical arrows* show the lateral masses and *horizontal arrow* shows the midline.

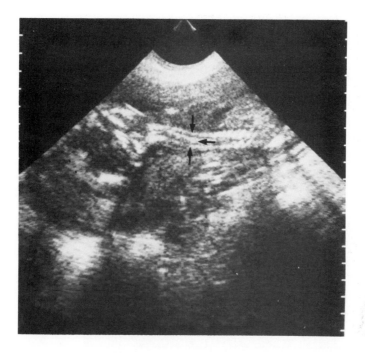

two atria, and the atrioventricular valves can usually be obtained in the second trimester. The septum primum, a thin membrane lying on the left side of the foramen ovale, is an important landmark (Figure 29). It has a biphasic valve-like motion and identifies the left atrium and the left-sided atrioventricular valves. Since fetal blood flows from the right atrium to the left atrium across the foramen ovale, this structure orients the observer to intracardiac anatomy. In addition, the right atrium can often be identified by the entrance of the inferior vena cava just above the confluence of the hepatic veins (Figure 30). The right ventricle can be distinguished from the left ventricle by its heavier trabeculation. In addition to the two atrioventricular valves, the aortic and pulmonary valves can also be identified, and the continuity of the aortic with the left-sided atrioventricular (mitral) valve is an important sign of a normal heart (Figure 31). The inferior vena cava, aortic arch, brachycephalic vessels, and descending aorta and iliac vessels are all well visualized with high quality real-time equipment.

Arrhythmias

Normal second trimester fetuses are often observed to have a transient bradycardia to 60 without

Figure 22

Widening of the laminae in the lumbar region in a longitudinal scan through the spine.

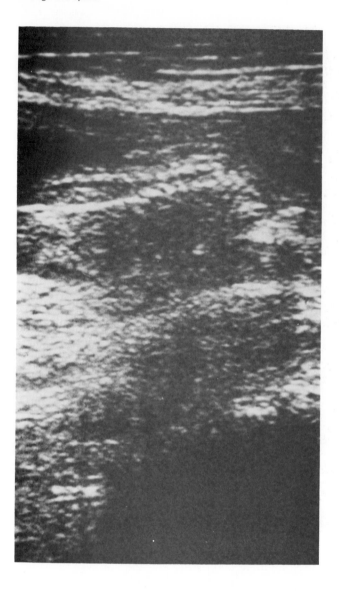

consequence. An occasional third trimester fetus will have a sustained bradycardia from atrioventricular block resulting from structural abnormalities or maternal connective tissue disease. We have recently studied 44 fetuses with echocardiography who had disturbances of cardiac rhythms (24):

Two fetuses with atrial flutter were hydropic. One responded to immediate delivery and cardioversion; the other did not. Three fetuses with potentially lethal

Figure 23

Short-axis section through the upper lumbar spine at 23 weeks. *Arrows* point to laminae.

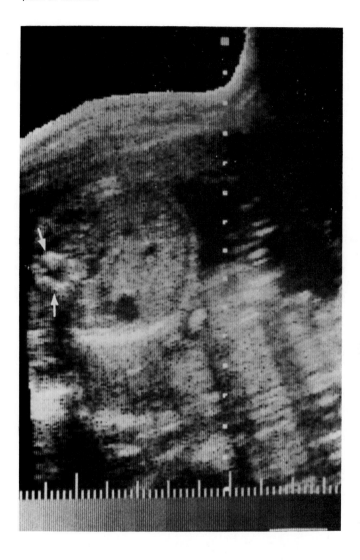

dysrhythmias were treated by maternal administration of digitalis. In each case the fetal heart rates were normalized. It has, therefore, been demonstrated that in utero treatment of some severe, life-threatening rhythm disturbances is possible (Table 1).

Structural abnormalities of the heart

Cardiac anomalies diagnosed in utero include endocardial cushion defect (often associated with trisomy 21), tetralogy of Fallot, hypoplastic or single ventricle, atrioventricular valve atresia, and interseptal rhabdomyoma. In some cases the defect can be

Figure 24

Transverse scan through lumbar spine at 23½ weeks showing typical wedge-shaped divergence of laminae.

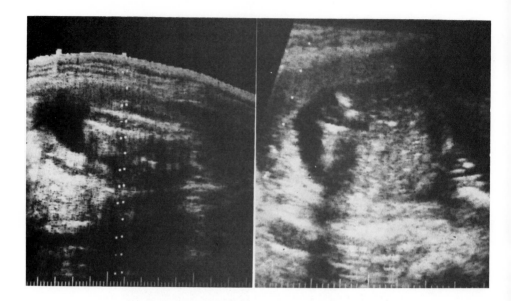

assessed to be surgically correctable. In other cases, such as hypoplastic left heart, the prognosis is hopeless. This knowledge is invaluable in planning obstetrical management.

The fetal heart is now such a rich source of information it is impossible to do justice to the subject in a review chapter on normal and abnormal fetal anatomy. In view of the rapid progress being made in fetal echocardiography it is likely that a whole chapter will be devoted to this subject in the next edition of this book.

Abdomen

Although the fetal abdomen is examined routinely and measurements of abdominal perimeter are used to estimate fetal weight, anatomical landmarks are often ignored. Since the umbilical vein is mainly cephalocaudal in direction, it does not accurately define a transverse cross section of the abdomen (Figure 32). On the other hand, the confluence of the umbilical vein with the portal sinus is an excellent marker of a true transverse cross section of the fetal abdomen because the portal sinus is directed posteriorly to the right side of the fetus (29, 30) (Figure 33). The fetal gallbladder is found at the bisection of

Figure 25

Transverse scan through sacral spine (*thin arrows*) showing protuberant meningomyelocele (*curved open arrow*). *Heavy white arrow* points to umbilical vein.

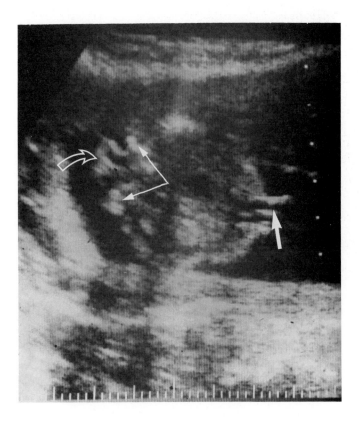

the angle between these two vessels (Figure 34). The ductus venosus is a cephalic continuation of the umbilical vein, but it is considerably narrower and joins the vena cava near the confluence of the hepatic veins just before the cava enters the right atrium (Figure 35). The fetal stomach, on the left side of the fetal abdomen, is always filled with fluid unless there is esophageal atresia without a fistula (Figure 36). The degree of gastric distention is, however, variable. In polyhydramnios the fetus apparently attempts to diminish the intrauterine volume by swallowing up to 700 cc of amniotic fluid a day (12). The stomach almost always appears to be quite full in normal fetuses with polyhydramnios (Figure 37). Prominent bowel loops are often noticed in normal term fetuses. This finding, however, is very unusual in premature fetuses (less than 36 weeks' gestation). *Markedly* dilated loops of bowel do not represent a normal variant at any time in gestation.

Figure 26

Coronal section through fetal body. *Arrows* show diaphragm; heart and left lung are shown. *L,*

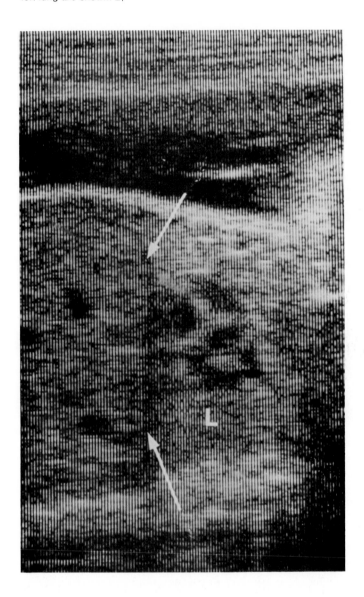

Abnormalities of abdominal wall

> Defects of the abdominal wall are of two types, gastroschisis and omphalocele. Gastroschisis occurs in 1:20,000 live births (Figure 38). The term is a misnomer in that the lesion has nothing to do with the stomach. It is a fusion defect that may involve the thorax and is rarely larger than 3 to 5 cm. Abdominal viscera herniate through the defect and are not covered by peritoneal membranes. The umbilicus is intact and inserts at its normal site. Obstruction due to atresia

Figure 27

Bilateral pleural effusion at 32 weeks. *Curved arrows* show pleural effusion above diaphragm.

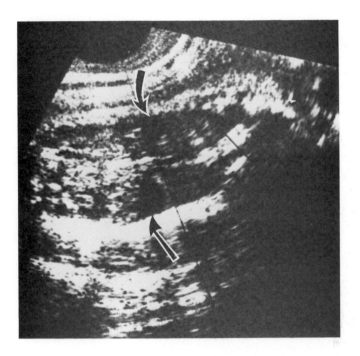

Figure 28a

Sagittal scan of a fetus in vertex presentation. Notice the presence of hydramnios and echo-spared areas in the fetal chest and abdomen. This fetus had duodenal atresia and an associated diaphragmatic hernia.

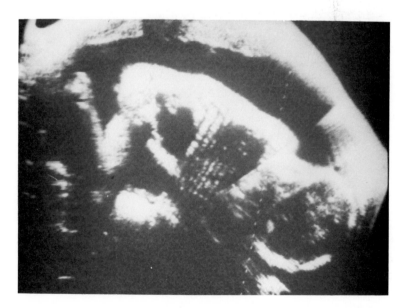

Figure 28b

Transverse scan through the diaphragm of the same fetus. Notice the large defect.

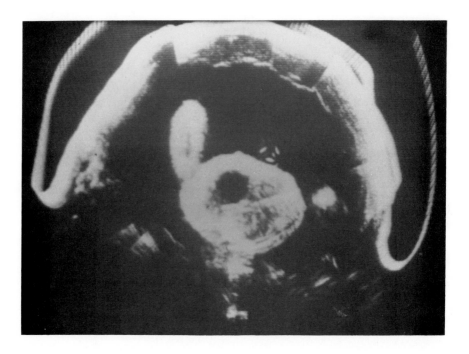

Figure 29

Coronal section through the fetal heart. *r*, right ventricle; *l*, left ventricle; *curved arrow* points to septum primum which lies to the left of the foramen ovale.

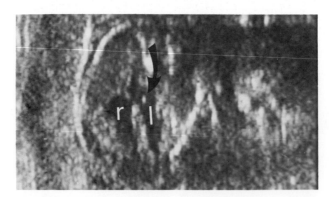

may be present, and since the bowel is freely floating in amniotic fluid one can readily observe loops of bowel and the pulsation of the mesenteric vessels (13). Serial scans are useful in monitoring the status of the lesion

Figure 30

Longitudinal scan showing inferior vena cava (*open curved arrow*)
entering right atrium (*closed curved arrow*).

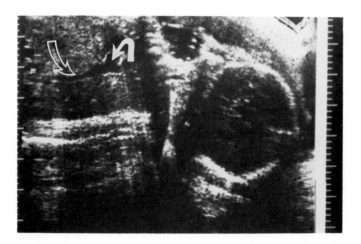

Figure 31

On the *left* the aortic root (*arrows*) and aortic valve are seen. On the
right the anterior leaf of the mitral valve is shown (*arrow*) and is
continuous with the posterior aortic root.

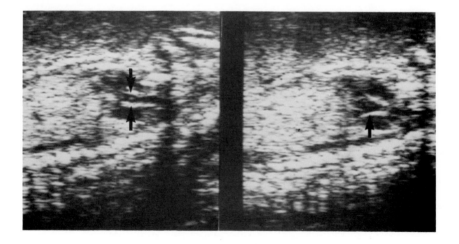

with regard to the extent of bowel obstruction and
presence of perforation. In fact, the timing of delivery
may depend very heavily upon ultrasound information.

Omphalocele results from a defect in the umbilical ring
with herniation of liver or bowel. It occurs in 1:6000 live
births. The extruded viscera are covered with a

Table 1
Summary of clinical data in 13 consecutive fetuses with non-immune hydrops*

Case No.	Gestation (wk)	Presenting Problem	Prenatal Diagnosis	Outcome and Pathological Findings
1	32	Polyhydramnios	Hydrops fetalis Intracardiac tumor	Stillbirth (33 weeks) Septal rhabdomyoma
2	28	Polyhydramnios	Hydrops fetalis Isolated levocardia Situs inversus Complete heart block Atrioventricular-canal defect	Premature birth (34 weeks) Complete heart block Death at 10 min. of life Isolated levocardia, situs inversus, polysplenia, atrioventricular-canal defect
3	28	Irregular fetal cardiac rhythm (Polyhydramnios)	Hydrops fetalis Complex dysrhythmia Tetralogy of Fallot Congestive cardiomyopathy	Cesarean delivery (31 weeks) Tetralogy of Fallot Ventricular dysrhythmia Congestive cardiomyopathy Hyaline membrane disease Death at 5 days
4	32	Polyhydramnios	Placental hydrops Right ventricular and right atrial dilatation Pulmonary stenosis ? Pulmonary insufficiency	Premature birth (33 weeks) "Absent pulmonary valve" syndrome; interventricular septum intact Hyaline membrane disease Death at 1 day
5†	38	Polyhydramnios	Hydrops fetalis Atrial flutter with 2:1 atrioventricular block	Cesarean delivery (38 weeks) Atrial flutter with 2:1 atrioventricular block Cardioversion (direct current) Survival in good condition
6	34	Polyhydramnios	Hydrops fetalis Atrial flutter with 5:1 and 6:1 atrioventricular block	Stillbirth (34 weeks) Dilated, anatomically normal heart
7	27	Irregular fetal cardiac rhythm	Pericardial effusion Supraventricular ectopy leading to paroxysmal atrial tachycardia	Transplacental digoxin therapy leading to sinus rhythm Delivery at 39 weeks Chaotic atrial rhythm treated with digoxin and propranolol Survival in good condition
8	36	Polyhydramnios	Twin pregnancy Twin A—"acardiac" monster Twin B—hydrops fetalis	Premature delivery Twin A—stillbirth and dysmorphism Twin B—hydrops, hyaline membrane disease, disseminated intravascular coagulation; death at 3 days
9	32	Polyhydramnios	Hydrops fetalis Normal heart	Stillbirth (33 weeks) Cystic adenomatoid malformation of right lung
10	29	Polyhydramnios	Hydrops fetalis Mediastinal mass Normal heart	Stillbirth (29 weeks) Extralobar sequestration Normal heart
11	22	Polyhydramnios	Hydrops fetalis Normal heart Abnormal chromosome No. 11	Premature birth (28 weeks) Respiratory distress Death at 30 min. of life Multiple anomalies

Table—*continued*

Case No.	Gestation (wk)	Presenting Problem	Prenatal Diagnosis	Outcome and Pathological Findings
12	32	Polyhydramnios	Hydrops fetalis Large ventricular septal defect	Diaphragmatic hernia Hypoplastic lungs Bilateral hydroureter Premature delivery Asplenia, atrial isomerism, atrioventricular-canal defect, transposition of great arteries, pulmonary atresia, anomalous pulmonary venous drainage Death at 3 days
13	33	Polyhydramnios	Hydrops fetalis Dilated atrium and ventricle	Premature delivery Death at 30 min. of life Dilated left atrium and ventricle Coronary artery embolus with massive myocardial infarction

* From Kleinman et al. (23).
† This case has been previously described by Kleinman, C.S., Hobbins, J.C., Jaffe, C.C., Lynch D.C., Talner, N.S.: Echocardiographic studies of the human fetus: prenatal diagnosis of congenital heart disease and cardiac dysrhythmias. Pediatrics 65:1059, 1980.

reflected peritoneal membrane, and the umbilical vessels are seen to enter the periabdominal mass (Figure 39). Unlike gastroschisis, fetuses with an omphalocele have a higher risk of associated anomalies of the cardiovascular system (16 to 20%), genitourinary system (40%), and central nervous system (4%) (34). Furthermore, approximately 30% have an associated chromosomal abnormality which is detectable by karyotype. Complications involving the gastrointestinal system can be present, such as atresia of the bowel (secondary to vascular compromise), incomplete rotation of the intestine, and, occasionally, abnormal fixation of the liver (34). The mortality rate varies between 20 and 30% and is due to infection, inanition, or unrelated congenital anomalies.

In both ventral wall defects prenatal diagnosis can be lifesaving for the fetus since it allows timely delivery in a hospital where pediatric surgeons can repair the defect promptly. Such management has recently been shown to improve survival rates. Also, since new MSAFP screening programs are rapidly being initiated, many more patients whose fetuses have ventral wall defects will be sent for ultrasound evaluation (20). The wary operator, realizing that AFP may leak into the amniotic cavity through an abdominal wall defect, should closely scrutinize the fetal cord insertion and nearby areas in these patients.

Figure 32

Aborted fetus injected with barium through the umbilical vein (*uv*). *PS*, portal sinus; *PV*, portal vein; IVC, inferior vena cava; *dv*, ductus venosus.

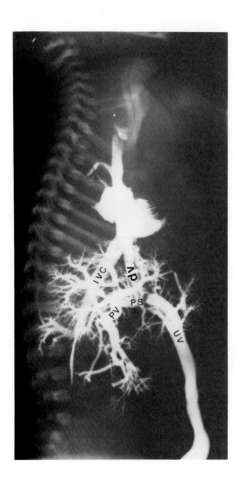

Gastrointestinal tract obstruction

Inability to visualize the fetal stomach with ultrasound should lead one to suspect esophageal atresia, but in most cases of atresia a tracheoesophageal fistula allows the stomach to fill with fluid. The so-called "double bubble" sign is indicative of duodenal atresia (Figure 40) which is frequently associated with trisomy 21 (19), but any fixed dilated segment of gut should lead to the consideration of obstructing lesions of the small bowel, particularly if associated with hydramnios. Duodenal obstruction may also occur with malrotation and annular pancreas. Distal obstructions are more difficult to recognize since they are not usually associated with hydramnios, but even anal atresia has been diagnosed in utero (1).

Figure 33

Transverse section through fetal abdomen. The spine is casting an acoustic shadow; umbilical vein (*small arrow*); portal sinus (*open arrow*).

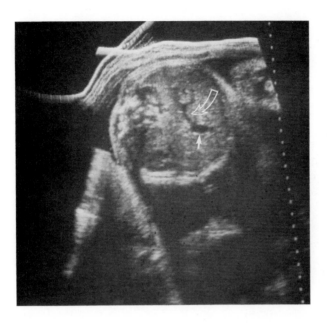

The syndromes reported thus far in the literature that have been associated with dilated bowel detected in utero are meconium ileus (19), "apple peel" atresia of the small bowel (10), jejunal atresia (25), megacystic-microcolon intestinal hypoperistalsis syndrome (6, 41), and intestinal aganglionosis involving the colon and distal ileum (43).

We have had the occasion to diagnose two cases of cystic fibrosis in utero based on ultrasound findings compatible with meconium ileus (Figure 41). In one fetus followed with daily ultrasound scanning it was possible to diagnose visceral perforation when ascites occurred. This was confirmed following emergency cesarean section. In the second case the couple had previously delivered a baby with cystic fibrosis and had prenatal testing in the second trimester. The amniotic fluid analysis for MUGB (methyl umbelliferyl guanidino benzoate) suggested a normal fetus. However, a third trimester scan revealed multiple loops of bowel that were first prominent and later dilated and filled with particulate matter. The infant has cystic fibrosis.

Fetal ascites, due to either hydrops or urinary tract obstruction, is readily seen (Figure 42). Massive

Figure 34

Cross section of fetal abdomen showing gallbladder (*arrows*).

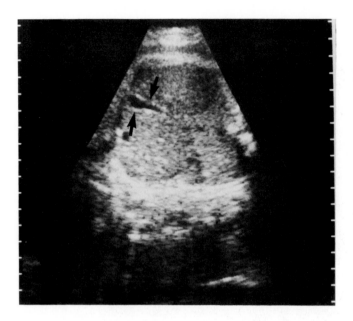

dilatation of the bladder displacing the liver must be distinguished from peritoneal fluid that surrounds the liver and divides the anatomical right and left lobes. There is a normal thin sonolucent band around the abdomen that may be due to a small normal quantity of peritoneal fluid or an acoustic artifact (pseudoascites) (Figures 36 and 37). Liquid-containing abdominal masses include mesenteric cysts, physiological ovarian cysts in female fetuses, teratomas, and choledochal cysts.

Genitourinary system

The fetal kidneys are seen beginning at about 16 weeks. They have more prominent renal pyramids than adult kidneys and the renal sinus contains little fat and is not strongly echogenic. In general, the two kidneys on cross section should not occupy more than one-third of the total abdominal area (Figure 43). This relationship can be numerically expressed by means of the mean kidney circumference-to-abdominal circumference (KC/AC) ratio. Grannum et al. have found that a ratio of 0.30 is constant throughout pregnancy with normal kidneys (15). With high resolution ultrasound it is possible to identify arcuate arteries, separating columns, and, often, individual calyces. Minimal dilation of the renal pelvis with

Figure 35

Ductus venosus (*arrow heads*) joining inferior vena cava (*ivc*) just before entering right atrium (*h*).

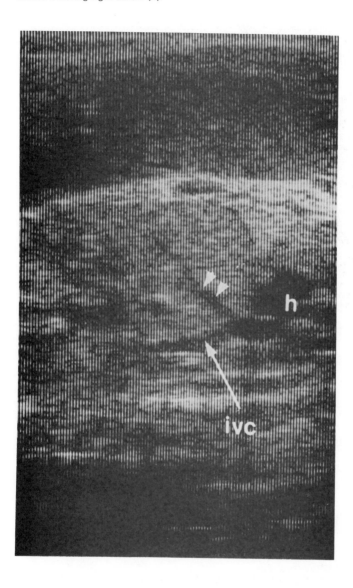

calyectasis is a normal finding. Under normal circumstances the ureter should not be visualized, but the bladder always can be identified, even shortly after the fetus voids. It is our impression that the bladder never completely empties when the fetus voids, a phenomenon that occurs about every 60 to 90 min. In a small fetus (less than 18 weeks) it is possible to miss the fetal bladder, but certainly if one cannot identify a bladder on two successive examinations within an hour (especially if there is oligohydramnios) one should

Figure 36

Transverse scan through fetal abdomen showing normal stomach (s).
Arrow points to spine.

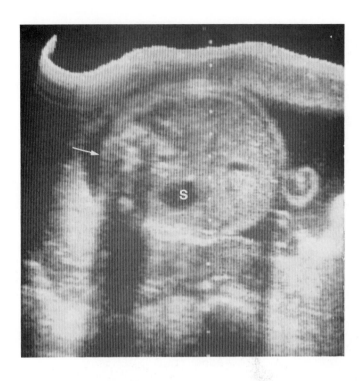

Figure 37

Longitudinal section through a fetus with hydramnios. The stomach (s)
is moderately dilated. *h*, heart.

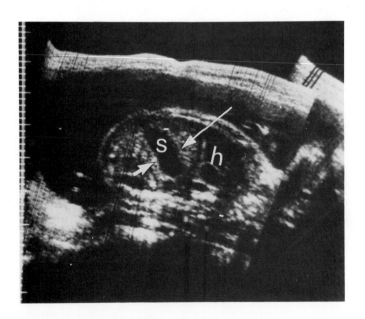

Figure 38a

Transverse scan showing bowel (*B*) protruding from the abdomen in a fetus with gastroschisis. Notice that the bowel is not surrounded by peritoneum.

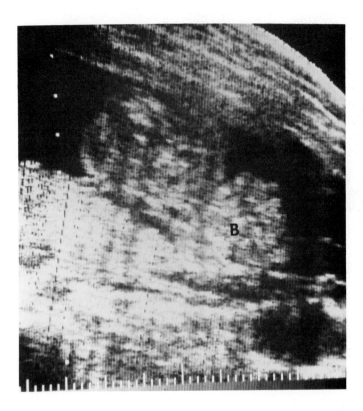

strongly suspect non-functioning kidneys. The urethra should never be seen in normal circumstances.

Some investigators have advocated the use of frusemide to stimulate fetal diuresis (42). This drug works best after the 20th week of gestation when the kidney tubules begin to function.

There are approximately 200 anomalies of the genitourinary system (2). Although Potter syndrome was originally described in infants with renal agenesis, the classic Potter's phenotype of pulmonary hypoplasia, blunted facies, and arthrogrypotic limbs can occur with any renal abnormality in which oligohydramnios is a feature. The incidence of renal agenesis is between 1 and 3 per 1,000. In this condition it is almost impossible to directly demonstrate absence of the kidneys because profound oligohydramnios prevents adequate visualization. Furthermore, the fetal adrenals may enlarge and

Figure 38b

Dilated loop of bowel (*b*) in amniotic fluid. *T*, trunk.

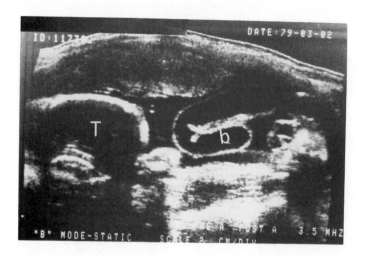

assume a reniform shape in the absence of the kidneys (Figure 44). Therefore, the diagnosis is based on the presence of marked oligohydramnios and an inability to demonstrate a fetal bladder (23).

Infantile polycystic kidney disease is an autosomal recessive condition with a 25% recurrence rate. It is uniformly lethal, with neonates dying of pulmonary hypoplasia. The term "polycystic" is inappropriate to describe the ultrasound findings since the kidneys are filled with microscopic cysts and appear to be solidly enlarged (Figure 45). In our experience the kidneys may not be discernibly enlarged until after the 20th week of gestation when they can triple in size in a 2-week period. Moreover, the oligohydramnios classically observed at birth may not be apparent until after the 20th week of gestation. By the 24th week of gestation, however, most polycystic kidneys should be ultrasonically detectable.

Multicystic kidney disease is generally unilateral and not lethal if one kidney is functioning (16) (Figure 46). It has a low recurrence rate. The cysts in the dysplastic (multicystic) kidneys are generally peripheral compared with the multiple dilated renal calyces and pelvis resulting from urinary tract obstruction. A unilateral multicystic kidney does not require intervention since the cysts atrophy and calcify in adulthood.

The urinary tract can be obstructed at any level. Ureteropelvic junction (UPJ) obstruction is generally

Figure 39

Transverse scan of a fetus with an omphalocele containing a portion of the fetal liver. *Large white arrow*, abdomen; *thin arrow*, omphalocele; *small arrow*, umbilical vein.

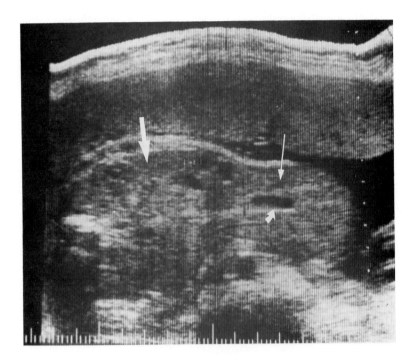

unilateral. The dilated renal pelvis often resembles a solitary cyst. Expectant management is advocated since the lesion is compatible with life. Occasionally, polyhydramnios can occur if the dilated kidney obstructs venous return or interferes with gastrointestinal absorption. Recently, we have diagnosed a unilateral ureteral obstruction in association with a type II dysplastic kidney.

A posterior urethral valve is a membrane that develops in the urethra and partially or completely obstructs the flow of urine. They occur only in male fetuses and are so thin that they are often missed in utero (Figure 47). While the "classical" picture of urethral obstruction includes a grossly dilated bladder and bilateral hydroureters and hydronephrosis (33), this is not always the case. Bladder outlet obstruction early in gestation may result in a constellation of findings which has been called the urethral obstruction malformation complex. This includes dystrophic muscular changes in the abdominal wall (prune belly syndrome) (6) (Figure 48), cryptorchidism (obstructed descent of testes secondary to the massively dilated bladder), absence of the mesocolon and/or malrotation of the colon

Figure 40

Scan through fetal abdomen showing distended stomach and duodenum.

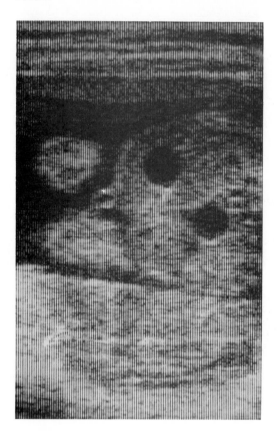

Figure 41

Longitudinal scan through a fetus with meconium ileus showing multiple loops of dilated bowel.

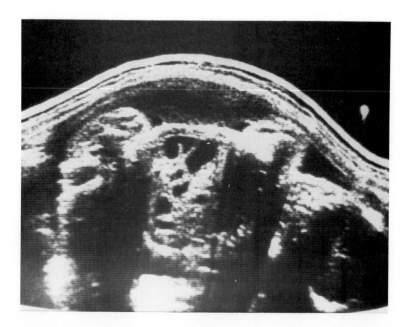

Figure 42
Longitudinal scan of a fetus with erythroblastosis fetalis. Ascites surrounds the bladder. The liver is markedly enlarged. Edema of the abdominal wall is also evident.

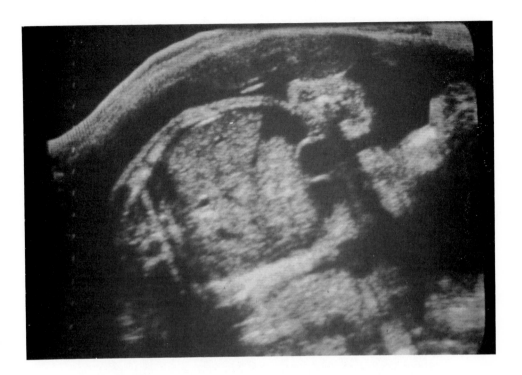

(prevention of gut rotation and fixation of the dorsal mesentery by the large bladder), and skeletal anomalies (oligohydramnios causing compression, abdominal distention causing rib deformities, and iliofemoral arterial compression). When the obstruction is incomplete, none of these findings may be present. Furthermore, hydronephrosis may be minimal or only unilateral in this condition. This is probably due to incompetence and reflux at only one ureteral orifice.

It must be remembered that oligohydramnios is not always the rule in urinary tract obstruction. Combinations of urinary and intestinal obstruction may tilt the balance in the direction of polyhydramnios. (We have seen one case of hypoganglionosis and dysplastic kidney with hydramnios, and dysplastic kidneys associated with hydramnios have been reported in the literature (Figure 49).)

If an abnormality that is compatible with extrauterine life is detected in utero, the fetus should be carefully followed. Apparent hydronephrosis has been seen to disappear spontaneously, and unilateral ureteropelvic

Figure 43

Transverse section through fetal abdomen with the fetus lying prone.
Both normal kidneys (*L* and *R*) are seen adjacent to the spine (*black
arrow*), which is casting an acoustic shadow (*open arrow*). *s*, stomach.

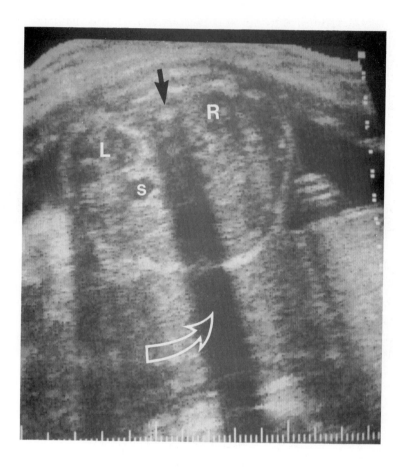

obstruction can await delivery before intervention
(Figure 50). Despite the complexity of renal lesions
there are two simple but important functional findings,
the presence of urine in the bladder and an adequate
quantity of amniotic fluid. If both of these are present in
the third trimester, the probability of lethal kidney
disease is remote.

Fetal limbs

In most cases it is possible to measure fetal long
bones. The most accessible bone is the femur, which
usually lies at an angle of 30° to 70° with the long axis
of the fetal body (Figure 51). The humerus is somewhat
more difficult to image and is often almost parallel with

Figure 44

Transverse scan through a fetus with renal agenesis and severe oligohydramnios. The fetal adrenals are visible and could be mistaken for kidneys.

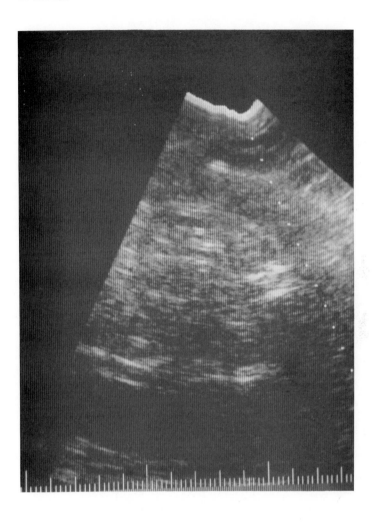

the fetal body. Since the fetal limbs are often in motion, the best way to measure long bones is with real-time. The easiest technique is to find one end of the bone to be evaluated and to fan the transducer in an arc until all of the bone is in one frozen image. We recommend that many images be obtained and that the longest consistent measurements be recorded, since there is a great tendency to obtain tangential cuts which results in falsely shortened measurements. It is reassuring to see a flared or rectangular rather than a pointed bone end (Figure 52). The latter suggests foreshortening due to obliquity. On the other hand, it is virtually impossible to "overshoot" on measurements of long bones unless

Figure 45

Enlarged kidney in 23-week fetus with classic infantile polycystic kidneys.

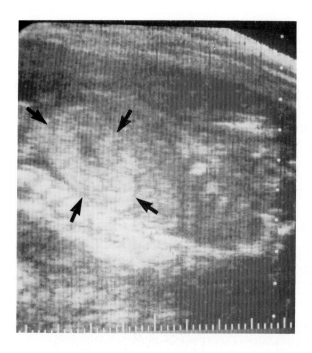

one erroneously incorporates an adjacent bone into the measurement. Since the cartilaginous ends of these bones are not densely echogenic, there is always an acoustic hiatus across a joint. In fact, this phenomenon is responsible for discrepancies in ultrasound measurements of long bones of abortuses in a water bath when compared with those made externally with a plastic rule (17), but measurements of diaphyseal length with ultrasound and radiography show excellent correlation.

Fetal femur and humerus length increase linearly until the mid-third trimester when there is some tailing off of incremental growth. As mentioned earlier, some authors have advocated the use of femur length as a predictor of gestational age since standard deviations are comparable (and in one study narrower) at each gestational age to those of BPD. This is surprising since in our opinion measurements of the long bones are more difficult than that of the BPD.

Skeletal dysplasias

More than 40 skeletal dysplasias have been described, many of which can be diagnosed with ultrasound in the

Figure 46

Transverse scan showing a large unilateral multicystic kidney (*white arrows*). *Black arrows* point to normal kidney.

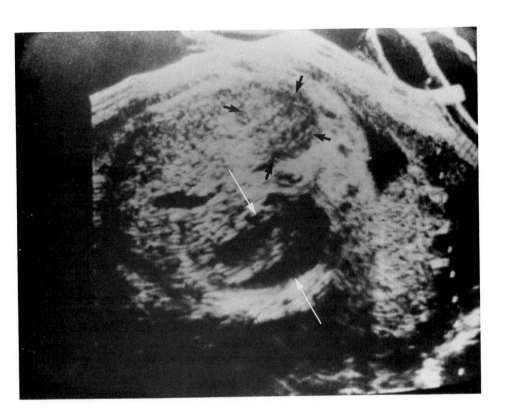

second trimester. All should be apparent in the late third trimester (37). Thus far, the conditions that have been diagnosed in the second trimester with ultrasound include homozygous achondroplasia (26), camptomelic dysplasia (17), diastrophic dysplasia (Figure 53*a* and *b*) (17, 27), osteogenesis imperfecta (autosomal dominant) (5), thrombocytopenia absent radii (TAR) syndrome (17), achondrogenesis (39), tetraphocomelia (Robert syndrome) (17), and an unclassified dysplasia (17).

Although accurate long bone measurements can be obtained in almost every fetus that can be plotted against standard nomograms for femur length, many more patients must be studied before it is possible to determine the sensitivity and specificity of this method in detecting specific conditions. For example, in two of our cases of the autosomal dominant variant of osteogenesis imperfecta, femur lengths in the second trimester were small but not outside 95% confidence limits. The diagnosis was possible in one case,

Figure 47

Twenty-four-week male fetus with posterior urethral valve partially
obstructing the bladder (*B*). The dilated urethra (*u*) and the valve itself
are seen.

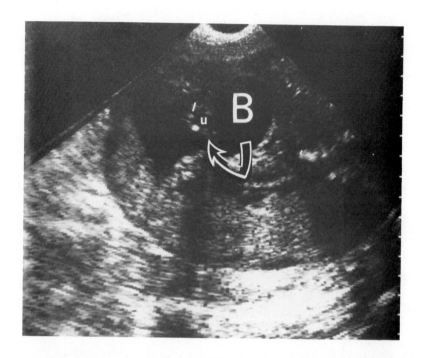

however, because an overriding fracture was noticed,
and in the second a dumbbell-like configuration of one
of the femurs was visualized. Later, the long bones
became ribbon-like and did not cast an acoustic
shadow because of poor mineralization. Therefore,
other features of a disease must be thoroughly
evaluated in addition to femur length. Also, in some
conditions such as heterozygous achondroplasia, long
bone length is not compromised until after 24 weeks of
gestation (9, 14).

Some skeletal dysplasias, although as yet not reported,
should be possible to diagnose in the second trimester
because of their severity at birth. These would include
osteogenesis imperfecta congenita (autosomal
recessive variant) (44), thanatophoric dysplasia (18),
and hypophosphatasia (31). All have been diagnosed in
the third trimester. In addition to examinations of the
long bones in certain skeletal dysplasias, it is useful to
evaluate other portions of the fetal anatomy that are
commonly affected. For example, a prominent forehead
is noted in achondroplasia and thanatophoric dysplasia.
A premaxillary protuberance is often observed in
Robert syndrome (19). "Hitchhiker thumbs" are a
feature of diastrophic dysplasia (27).

Figure 48

Sagittal scan demonstrating a dilated fetal bladder. At autopsy the bowel was compressed against the diaphragm.

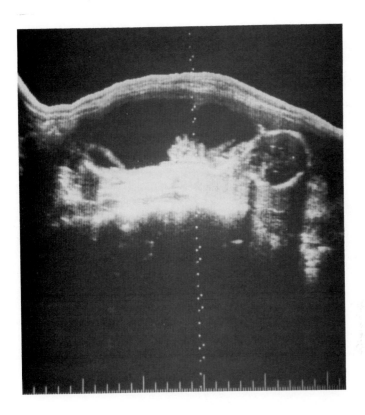

Figure 49

Massive distention of the bladder associated with hydramnios in a fetus with hypoganglionosis.

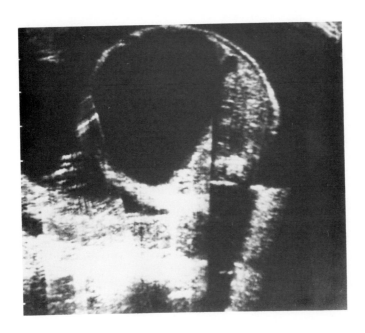

Figure 50

Moderate hydronephrosis in a fetus with incomplete urinary tract obstruction secondary to urethral valve.

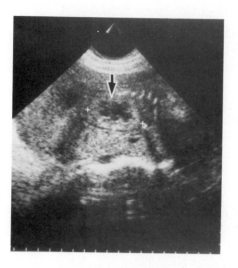

Figure 51

Schematic diagram showing the relationship of the femur to the aorta in the typical tucked position assumed by the fetus in utero.

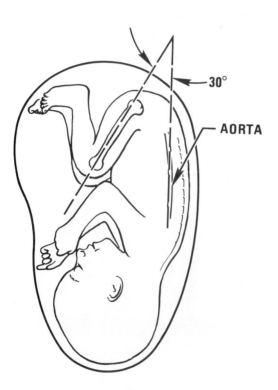

Figure 52

Linear array scan through both fetal femurs (*F*) at 23 weeks. Notice the flared ends of the upper femur, which is shown in its entirety.

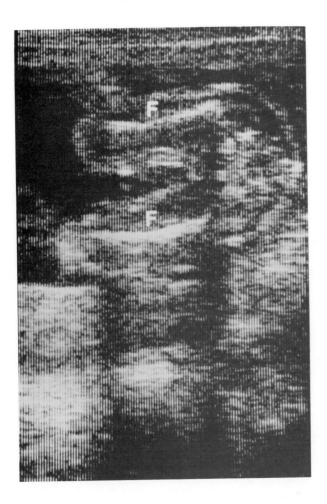

In the third trimester attempts should be made to specifically identify the type of dysplasia present, because obstetrical management may depend upon this diagnosis. For example, thanatophoric dysplasia is uniformly lethal. Knowing that a fetus has this condition, an obstetrician may elect not to deliver a patient by cesarean section if fetal distress is detected in labor.

The only practical importance of sex determination in the third trimester is that female fetuses with RDS respond better to steroid therapy than male fetuses. It is, however, often possible to visualize either the scrotum or penis in the period between the 16th and 20th week (Figure 54). At about the 26th week the

Figure 53

Scan through upper legs of a normal fetus (*a*) (11-14-79) and a fetus with diastrophic dysplasia (*b*) (10-19-79).

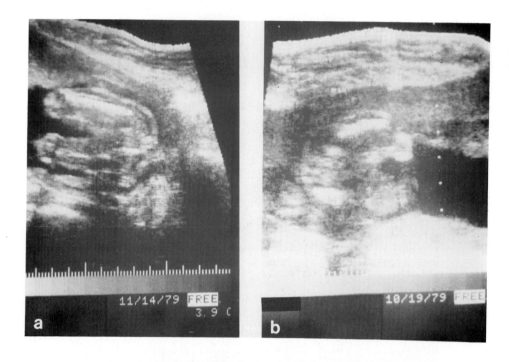

Figure 54

♂ Scrotum and penis of a male fetus at 34 weeks.

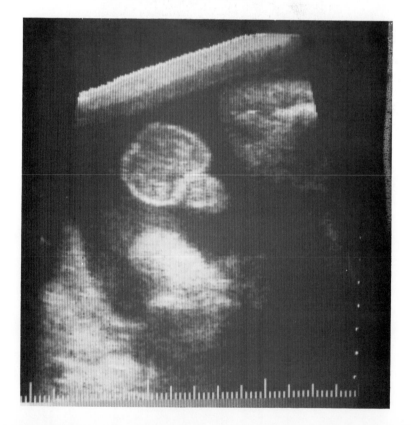

Figure 55

♀ The vulva of a female fetus at term.

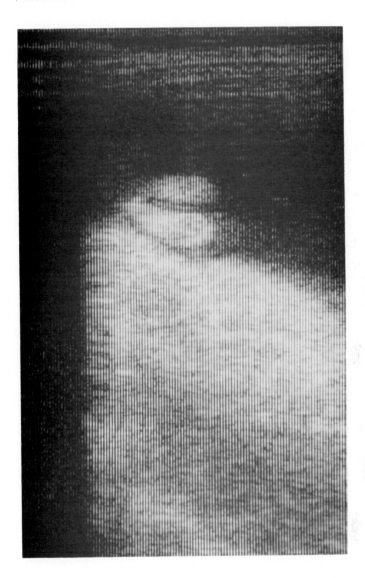

vulva and labia can be visualized (Figure 55), but
clitoral hypertrophy can be confused with a penis.

The normal umbilical cord containing two arteries and
one vein can be differentiated from the single artery
cord with ultrasound in the second trimester by
visualizing each of the vessels (Figure 56).
Furthermore, the normal cord has a braided
appearance in the second trimester, and when this is
observed a single artery can be excluded. As single
artery cords may be associated with a variety of
anomalies, this finding should alert the

Figure 56

Cross section through an umbilical cord showing two arteries and a vein.

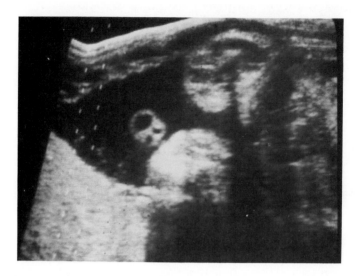

ultrasonographer to the possibility of other abnormalities.

Attachment of the cord to the fetus at the umbilicus and into the placenta is easily detectable. The umbilical vein can be followed into the liver and the arteries into the iliac arteries. Measurements of the blood flow in the umbilical vein with pulsed Doppler have been made, and these may provide valuable information regarding fetal well-being. They are best made in the fetal liver before the division into the portal sinus.

As real-time equipment improves, imaging of the fetus will be easier, but the problems confronting the examiner will be correspondingly more difficult. It is much more difficult to detect subtle abnormalities such as polydactyly than gross hydrocephalus or massive bladder enlargement. Thus, we can expect that the job of the ultrasonographer will become more, not less, difficult as the capabilities of scanners increase.

References

1 **Bean, W.J., Calonje, M.A., Aprill, C.N., Geshner, J.:** Anal atresia: A prenatal ultrasound diagnosis. J. Clin. Ultrasound 6:111, 1978.

2 **Bergsma, D (ed.):** *Birth Defects Compendium*, 2nd ed. Alan R. Liss, New York, 1979.

3 **Brock, D.J.H.:** Mechanisms by which amniotic fluid alpha-fetoprotein may be increased in fetal abnormalities. Lancet 2:345, 1976.

4 **Brock, D.J.H.:** The prenatal diagnosis of neural tube defects. Obstet. Gynecol. Surv. 31:32, 1976.

5 **Chervenak, F.A., Romero, R., Berkowitz, R.L., Mahoney, M.J., Tortora, M., Mayden, K., Hobbins, J.C.:** Antenatal sonographic findings of osteogenesis imperfecta. Am. J. Obstet. Gynecol. 143:228, 1982.

6 **Cooperberg, P.L., Romalis, G., Wright, V.:** Megacystis (prune-belly syndrome): Sonographic demonstration in utero. J. Can. Assoc. Radiol. 30:120, 1979.

7 **Crane, J.P.:** Familial congenital diaphragmatic hernia: Prenatal diagnostic approach and analysis of twelve families. Clin. Genet. 16:244, 1979.

8 **Denkhaus, H., Winsberg, F.:** Ultrasonic measurement of the fetal ventricular system. Radiology 131:781–787, 1979.

9 **Filly, R.A., Golbus, M.S., Carey, J.C., Hall, J.G.:** Short-limbed dwarfism: Ultrasonographic diagnosis by mensuration of fetal femoral length. Radiology 138:653, 1981.

10 **Fletman, D., McQuown, D., Kanchanapoom, V., Gyepes, M.T.:** ''Apple peel'' atresia of the small bowel: Prenatal diagnosis of the obstruction by ultrasound. Pediatr. Radiol. 9:118, 1980.

11 **Frigoletto, F.D., Jr., Birnholz, J.C., Driscoll, S.G., Finberg, W.J.:** Ultrasound diagnosis of cystic hygroma. Am. J. Obstet. Gynecol. 136:962, 1980.

12 **Gitlin, D., Kumate, J., Morales, S., Noriega, L., Arévalo, N.:** The turnover of amniotic fluid protein in the human conceptus. Am. J. Obstet. Gynecol. 113:632, 1972.

13 **Giulian, B.B., Alvear, D.T.:** Prenatal ultrasonographic diagnosis of fetal gastroschisis. Radiology 129:473, 1978.

14 **Golbus, M.S., Hall, B.D.:** Failure to diagnose achondroplasia in utero. Lancet 1:629, 1974.

15 **Grannum, P., Bracken, M., Silverman, R., Hobbins, J.C.:** Assessment of fetal kidney size in normal gestation by comparison of ratio of kidney circumference to abdominal circumference. Am. J. Obstet. Gynecol. 136:249, 1980.

16 **Henderson, S.C., Van Kolken, R.J., Rahatzad, M.:** Multicystic kidney with hydramnios. J. Clin. Ultrasound 8:249, 1980.

17 **Hobbins, J.C., Bracken, M.B., Mahoney, M.J.:** Diagnosis of fetal skeletal dysplasia with ultrasound. Am. J. Obstet. Gynecol. 142:306, 1982.

18 **Hobbins, J.C., Mahoney, M.J.:** The diagnosis of skeletal dysplasias with ultrasound. In *The Principles and Practices of Ultrasonography in Obstetrics and Gynecology*, R.C. Sanders, A.E. James, ed., 2nd ed. Appleton-Century-Crofts, New York, 1980.

19 **Hobbins, J.C., Mahoney, M.J., Berkowitz, R.L., Grannum, P., Silverman, R.:** Ultrasound in the diagnosis of congenital anomalies. Am. J. Obstet. Gynecol. 134:331, 1979.

20 **Hobbins, J.C., Venus, I., Tortora, M., Mayden, K., Mahoney, M.J.:** Stage II ultrasound examination for the diagnosis of fetal abnormalities with an elevated amniotic fluid alpha-fetoprotein concentration. Am. J. Obstet. Gynecol. 142:1026, 1982.

21 **Holmes, L.B., Nash, A., ZuRhein, G.M., Levin, M., Opitz, J.M.:** X-linked aqueductal stenosis: Clinical and neuropathological findings in two families. Pediatrics 51:697, 1973.

22 **Johnson, M.L., Dunne, M.C., Mack, L.A., Rashbaum, C.L.:** Evaluation of fetal intracranial anatomy by static and realtime ultrasound. J. Clin. Ultrasound 8:311, 1980.

23 **Keirse, M.J., Meerman, R.H.:** Antenatal diagnosis of Potter syndrome. Obstet. Gynecol. 52:64s, 1978.

24 **Kleinman, C.S., Donnerstein, R.L., DeVore, G.R., Jaffe, C.C., Lynch, D.C., Berkowitz, R.L., Talner, N.H., Hobbins, J.C.:** Fetal echocardiography for evaluation of in utero congestive heart failure—a technique for study of non-immune fetal hydrops. N. Engl. J. Med. 306:568, 1982.

25 **Lee, T.G., Warren, B.H.:** Antenatal ultrasonic demonstration of fetal bowel. Radiology 124:471, 1977.

26 **Leonard, C.O., Sanders, R.C., Lau, H.L.:** Prenatal diagnosis of the Turner syndrome, a familial chromosomal rearrangement and achondroplasia by amniocentesis and ultrasonography. Johns Hopkins Med. J. 145:25, 1979.

27 **Mantagos, S., Weiss, R.R., Mahoney, M.J., Hobbins, J.C.:** Prenatal diagnosis of diastrophic dwarfism. Am. J. Obstet. Gynecol. 139:111, 1981.

28 **Mayden, K., Tortora, M., Bracken, M., Berkowitz, R.L., Hobbins, J.C.:** Orbital diameters—a new parameter for dating and prenatal diagnosis. Am. J. Obstet. Gynecol., in press.

29 **Morin, F.R., Winsberg, F.:** Ultrasound and radiographic study of the vessels of the fetal liver. J. Clin. Ultrasound 6:409–411, 1978.

30. **Morin, F.R., Winsberg, F.:** Ultrasonic appearance of the umbilical cord. J. Clin. Ultrasound. 6:324–326, 1978.

31 **Mulivor, R.A., Mennuti, M., Zackai, E.H., Harris, H.:** Prenatal diagnosis of hypophosphatasia: Genetic, biochemical, and clinical studies. Am. J. Hum. Genet. 30:271, 1978.

32 **Nevin, N.C., Thompson, W., Davison, G., Horner, W.T.:** Prenatal diagnosis of the Meckel syndrome. Clin. Genet. 15:1, 1979.

33 **Okulski, T.A.:** The prenatal diagnosis of lower urinary tract obstruction using B-scan ultrasound: A case report. J. Clin. Ultrasound 5:268, 1977.

34 **Pickett, L.K.:** Omphalocele. In *Birth Defects Compendium*, D. Bergsma, ed., 2nd ed. Alan R. Liss, New York, 1979, p. 807.

35 **Schulman, K.:** Anencephaly. In *Birth Defects Compendium*, D. Bergsma, ed., 2nd ed. Alan R. Liss, New York, 1979, p. 83.

36 **Shulman, K.:** Hydrocephaly. In *Birth Defects Compendium*, D. Bergsma, ed., 2nd ed. Alan R. Liss, New York, 1979, p. 534.

37 **Sillence, D.O., Rimoin, D.L., Lachman, R.:** Neonatal dwarfism: Symposium on medical genetics. Pediatr. Clin. North Am. 23:453, 1978.

38 **Smith, A.D., Wald, N.J., Cuckle, H.S., Stirrat, G.M., Borrow, M., Lagercrantz, H.:** Amniotic fluid acetylcholinesterase as a possible

diagnostic test for neural-tube defects in early pregnancy. Lancet 1:685, 1979.

39 **Smith, W.L., Breitweiser, T.D., Dinno, N.:** In utero diagnosis of achondrogenesis, Type I. Clin. Genet. 19:51, 1981.

40 **United Kingdom Collaborative Study on Alpha-fetoprotein in Relation to Neural Tube Defects :** Second report: Amniotic-fluid alpha-fetoprotein measurement in antenatal diagnosis of anencephaly and open spina bifida in early pregnancy. Lancet 2:651, 1979.

41 **Vezina, W.C., Morin, F. R., Winsberg, F.:** Megacystic-microcolon-intestinal hypoperistalsis syndrome: antenatal ultrasound appearance. Am J Radiology 133:749–750, 1979.

42 **Wladimiroff, J.W.:** Effect of frusemide on fetal urine production. Br. J. Obstet. Gynecol. 82:221, 1975.

43 **Wrobleski, D., Wesselhoeft, C.:** Ultrasonic diagnosis of prenatal intestinal obstruction. J. Pediatr. Surg. 14:598, 1979.

44 **Zervoudakis, I.A., Strongin, M.J., Schrotenboer, K.A., Behan, M., Kazam, E., Hawks, G.G.:** Diagnosis and management of fetal osteogenesis imperfecta congenita in labor. Am. J. Obstet. Gynecol. 131:1, 116, 1978.

Invasive Procedures

8

The information available from amniotic fluid (AF) analysis has been responsible for some of the most significant obstetrical advances in the past 20 years, but these advances depend upon our ability to obtain enough fluid to perform the necessary studies without harming the mother or fetus. A great deal of experience with amniocentesis has been amassed, and the risks, complications, and benefits of the technique are now fairly well-defined.

Reasons for performing amniocentesis

In the second trimester, amniotic fluid studies are usually performed for genetic indications. Desquamated fetal cells can be cultured in approximately 2 to 4 weeks. Chromosome studies, sex identification, enzyme analysis for a growing number of inborn errors of metabolism, and DNA restriction endonuclease studies can then be performed. In addition, cell-free amniotic fluid can be analyzed for specific substances such as alphafetoprotein, acetylcholinesterase, and some enzymes that are markers for specific fetal biochemical disorders. At the present time, information obtained from these studies is exclusively used to determine prognosis. The only option now available to a woman carrying a fetus who is affected with an inherited disorder is abortion, so that a diagnosis must be made during the time interval when therapeutic abortion is legally permitted. Ultimately, of course, we hope to be able to provide corrective therapy in utero to some affected infants, but this is not now possible.

In the third trimester, amniotic fluid studies are performed primarily to assess fetal well-being. Indices of fetal maturity are of particular importance since prematurity is the major cause of neonatal morbidity and mortality in North America today. Respiratory distress is the most significant problem of the premature neonate, so that indicators of pulmonic maturity are of greatest relevance prior to elective delivery. While the L/S (lecithin/sphingomyelin) ratio is most frequently used to predict pulmonic maturity, other tests include PG (phosphatidyl glycerol) analysis,

$\triangle OD_{650}$ studies, and the shake test. Since AF creatinine, orange cell counts, and bilirubin do not necessarily reflect fetal lung maturity, they are no longer widely used.

Photospectrometric analysis at 450 mμ ($\triangle OD_{450}$) reflects the quantity of indirect bilirubin present in AF. Serial determinations of this substance are the most accurate way to evaluate the extent of fetal compromise in Rh-sensitized pregnancies.

In patients at risk for amnionitis amniotic fluid is studied by gram stains to identify bacteria and/or white blood cells, and by culture and colony counts. White blood cells are not necessarily indicative of incipient amnionitis, but bacteria visible on the gram stain of an unspun specimen or colony counts in excess of 10^3 organisms/ml are probably diagnostic (4).

There is controversy about the significance of meconium in the AF in the management of pregnancies beyond 42 weeks. Moderate to severe postmaturity syndrome is always accompanied by the passage of meconium, and its presence in the amniotic fluid after 42 weeks suggests that dysmaturity may be present. Some authors maintain that serial electronic fetal heart rate testing is an acceptable alternative to weekly amniocentesis for meconium and avoids the morbidity associated with multiple taps (24), whereas others believe that heart rate changes may be relatively late signs of dysmaturity and are often preceded by the passage of meconium (2). As discussed in Chapter 4, "The placenta," grading of placental maturity may be very useful in diagnosing postmaturity.

Second trimester amniocentesis

Amniocentesis can be performed as early as the 14th week of gestation. It was initially believed that the earlier a genetic tap was performed the better, since a karyotype requires 14 to 24 days of cell culture growth. If the cells failed to grow, the amniocentesis would have to be repeated, followed by the same delay until karyotyping could be accomplished. In most cytogenetic tissue culture labs, however, it is rare for culture failures to occur; and if the cells are not thriving, this can be recognized within a few days of the tap. Amniocentesis is safer at about the 16th week of gestation, because there is more amniotic fluid (about 175 cc) (34) and consequently more options for tapping sites.

Method

Amniocentesis should be performed immediately following an ultrasound examination. Changes in

Figure 1a

Sagittal scan of an intrauterine pregnancy at 16 weeks with a full maternal bladder (*MB*). The placenta is anterior.

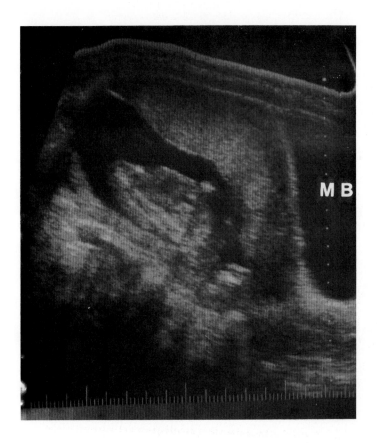

maternal bladder volume may significantly alter the relative positions of the placenta and anterior abdominal walls (16) (36) (Figure 1). Consequently, when a patient is scanned in one room and then moved to another for amniocentesis at a later time, the data from the initial scan are irrelevant. Furthermore, it is obvious that while intrinsic movement can always propel a fetus directly into a region chosen for needle insertion, the chances that this will occur increase with the interval between scan and tap, as well as with maternal movement.

Prior to performing a second trimester tap, ultrasonic assessment should include BPD measurement to verify gestational age, cardiac visualization with real-time to document life in utero, determination of fetal number and lie(s), and placental localization. After obtaining this information, a pocket of fluid should be sought which is not close to fetal vital parts and can be

Figure 1b

Sagittal scan of the same patient after the maternal bladder (*open arrow*) has been emptied. Notice that the uterus has rotated forward and an entry site for the amniocentesis needle at the fundus (*arrow*) has been revealed which will not necessitate penetrating the placenta.

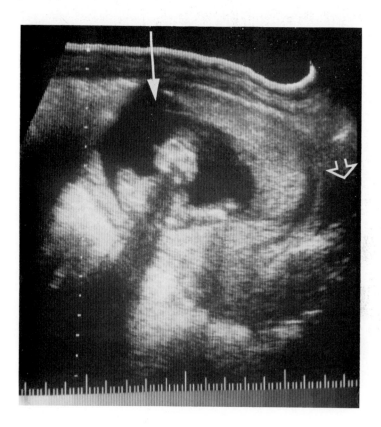

reached without penetrating the placenta (Figure 2). In about 40% of cases the placenta is implanted anteriorly, but the entire anterior surface of the uterus is not necessarily covered, and it is possible to find a placenta-free entry site in approximately half of these women. When placental penetration is unavoidable, it is preferable to traverse a peripheral extension rather than the thick central portion in order to reduce the risk of injuring large fetal vessels near the cord insertion (Figure 3). With static or real-time scanning, one can often locate the site of the placental cord insertion (Figure 4).

If a linear array is used to locate a pocket of amniotic fluid, the operator's finger should be inserted under the real-time head and slid along it until the finger's acoustic shadow is directly over the optimal site of entry (Figure 5). The skin on the patient's abdomen is

Figure 2

Sagittal scan showing a pocket of AF over a posterior placenta. Notice the shadows cast by the bones in the limb.

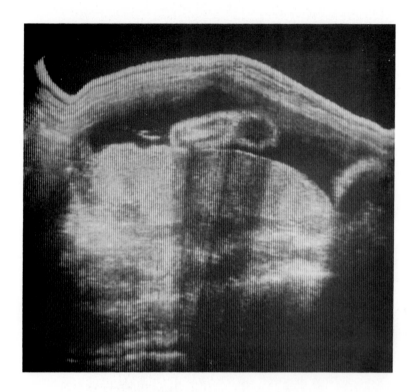

then marked by indentation at this point with the plastic hub of a disposable needle. If an articulated static scanner is used, the entry site, depth, and angle can be precisely pinpointed with the transducer itself. By displaying the graticule that shows the path of sound emitted by the transducer, the proposed path of the needle can be displayed from any spot on the maternal abdominal wall (Figure 6). Regardless of the type of scan performed, the last image produced before the tap should be left on the ultrasound screen to be used as a reference at the time of needle placement.

Since a potential source of morbidity is sepsis, it is imperative to maintain scrupulous aseptic technique. Non-sterile mineral oil should not be used prior to a tap unless it is removed with acetone. In most institutions it is impractical to follow the needle insertion with direct real-time visualization. If this is done, however, the insertion site must be protected from contamination. The real-time transducer should, therefore, either be gas-sterilized or placed in a sterile plastic bag prior to use. After the abdomen is prepared with an antiseptic

Figure 3

Graticule showing the path for needle insertion through the thin
portion of the anterior placenta.

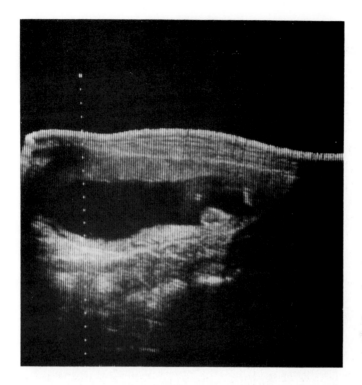

solution, the skin and subcutaneous tissues are
infiltrated with 3 cc of 1% lidocaine. Some operators do
not feel that infiltration with local anesthesia is
necessary and perform their taps without using it.

A 20- or 22-gauge disposable spinal tap needle with
central stylet measuring 9 cm from hup to tip is used in
most cases. In very obese patients a longer needle may
be required. When inserting the needle the operator
should feel each tissue layer as it is being penetrated.
Reference should be made to the displayed ultrasound
image in order to angle the needle properly and gauge
the depth of penetration. We have found it necessary to
advance the needle about 1 cm further than the actual
distance measured on the scan from skin surface to
midportion of the amniotic fluid pocket. This is difficult
to explain, but there are three possible reasons:

1   There is some compression of the skin by the
    transducer during the scan.
2   The skin tents up along the needle as it is inserted.
3   The local anesthesia increases the thickness of the
    tissue.

Figure 4

Sagittal scan showing the site of cord insertion in a pregnancy at 24 weeks.

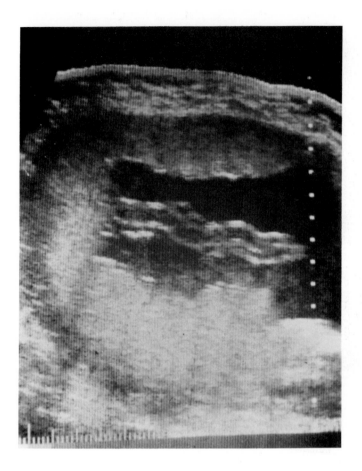

In any case, the stylet should be removed only when the desired distance is attained; then, if the cavity has been entered cleanly, clear fluid will usually appear at the needle hub.

If no fluid is obtained after the initial placement of the needle, it may be moved up or down along the axis of its introduction for 1 or 2 cm. Failure to enter a pocket of AF after performing these adjustments probably means that a contraction has occurred or the fetus has moved into the area of the tap. We recommend withdrawing the needle at this point and rescanning to find another entry site. Repeated blind thrusts of the needle or attempts to change its angle of introduction without visual reassessment are usually unsuccessful and may be dangerous for the fetus. If a second insertion is also unsuccessful, no further attempt should be made that day. The patient may be scheduled to return for another tap in 4 to 7 days.

Figure 5

The site of needle insertion for amniocentesis is marked by a shadow cast by the operator's finger under the linear array transducer in this scan.

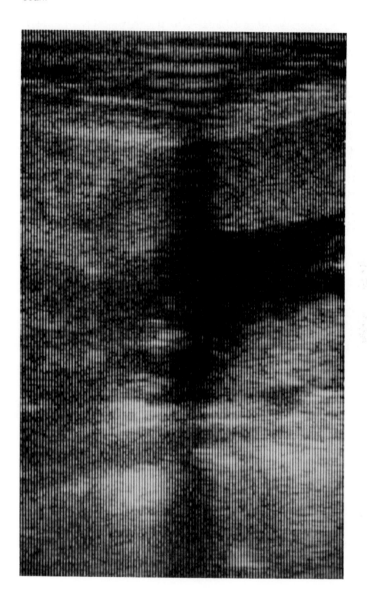

After a successful entry, the flow of fluid occasionally stops abruptly, possibly because negative pressure from the aspirating needle has pulled membranes, cord, or a portion of the fetus up against the bevel of the needle and occluded its opening. If this occurs, stop aspirating and simply rotate the needle 90 or 180° or gently massage the maternal abdomen. These maneuvers usually permit resumption of aspiration.

If the entry site into the amniotic sac is observed with real-time ultrasound immediately after withdrawing the

Figure 6

The graticule marks the path for needle insertion in this sagittal scan of a patient with a posterior placenta.

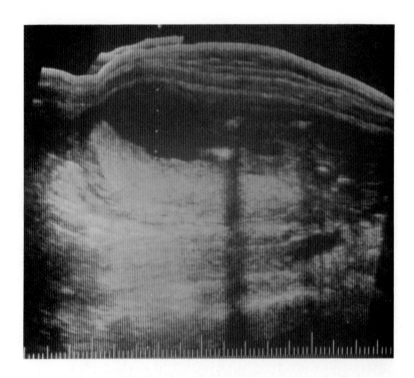

needle, a "shower" of blood may occasionally be seen. This is most likely to occur when an anterior placenta has been traversed. The ultrasonic picture is that of particulate matter moving through the AF and is caused by blood streaming down from the entry tract. Presumably, this bleeding has been temporarily tamponaded by the amniocentesis needle during the procedure. In our experience continued real-time observation invariably demonstrates the bleeding to stop within 30 to 60 sec.

Although real-time direct visualization of amniocentesis is not now a practical procedure in most hospitals, suitable instruments will probably be developed in the next few years. The use of direct visualization should further reduce the complications of genetic amniocentesis. Although we do not advocate the routine use of the A-mode aspiration transducer, one author (F.W.) uses it whenever the available space is small or intermittently occupied by the fetus, or after a dry tap.

A technique we have recently begun to use at Yale-New Haven Hospital is proving to be quite useful for

Figure 7

The tip of the amniocentesis needle can be visualized by real-time within the amniotic fluid.

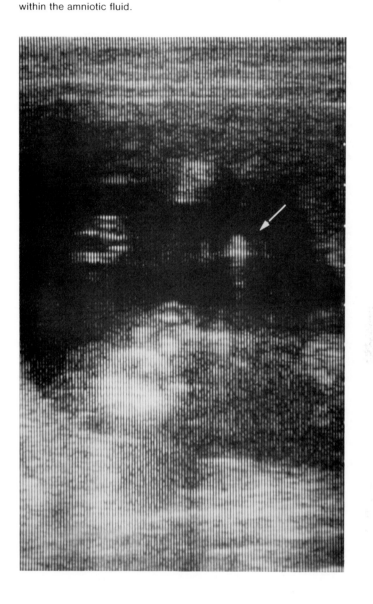

difficult taps. The real-time linear array transducer is placed in a sterile glove, and, after prepping the insertion site with Betadine, sterile contact gel is applied to the maternal abdomen. The insertion site is then visualized with the sterile-gloved transducer and the amniocentesis needle inserted parallel to and in contact with its side. The needle tip can subsequently be seen as a densely echogenic point traversing tissue layers and finally entering the pocket of fluid being tapped (Figure 7). If difficulty is encountered, the needle tip can be repositioned under direct real-time visualization.

Bloody taps and discolored amniotic fluid

Blood may interfere with cell growth in midtrimester amniocenteses. If the first 5 cc of fluid are bloody, another sample should be aspirated into a second syringe. If the fluid continues to be bloody, syringes should be changed until a clear specimen is obtained or 25 cc of fluid have been withdrawn. Even when an anterior placenta is penetrated, clear AF is usually obtained with the above technique, since blood clots rapidly on the placental surface. After obtaining 20 cc of clear fluid we suggest that the syringe be disengaged before the needle is removed from the abdomen, since myometrial blood can be inadvertently aspirated into the syringe as the needle is withdrawn.

Bloody taps containing significant quantities of fetal blood may have spuriously high levels of alphafetoprotein. Therefore, if AFP analysis is to be performed on a grossly bloody specimen of amniotic fluid, a Kleihauer-Betke stain should be done to measure the degree of fetal blood contamination. This test relies upon differences in the physical properties of adult and fetal hemoglobin. Treatment of a peripheral smear of the mother's blood with an acid solution selectively causes the elution of hemoglobin from her red blood cells. Subsequent staining of the smear reveals highly visible fetal cells against a background of maternal "ghost cells." By counting the number of fetal cells/1000 maternal red blood cells the degree of feto-maternal transfusion can be calculated.

We know from experience with placental aspiration that it is possible to obtain a large number of fetal red blood cells from a specimen of amniotic fluid without jeopardizing the fetus. Nevertheless, the amniocentesis needle can create a rent in a fetal vessel through which a significant quantity of blood may be lost. For this reason, it is wiser to perform a genetic tap at 16 weeks when 1 cc of fetal blood represents a 6% blood volume depletion than at 14 weeks when the same 1 cc blood loss represents a 15% fetal blood volume deficit.

If brown or darkly stained green fluid is obtained at the time of the tap, two possibilities must be considered. The discolored fluid may be the consequence of a fetal demise which occurred several days prior to the amniocentesis. This should have been diagnosed prior to amniocentesis by visualizing no fetal cardiac activity with the real-time scanner. Alternatively, the dark fluid may be secondary to hemoglobin breakdown products in a woman who has had some vaginal bleeding. This is probably due to the transudation of pigment from a retromembranous collection of blood. In one study six of 234 second trimester taps produced greenish fluid, and all pregnancies terminated in the birth of healthy children (21). In another report 10 of 514 taps produced dark fluid; three of these cases ended in fetal demise within 1 to 3 weeks, while the remaining seven pregnancies resulted in the delivery of normal neonates (23).

Twins

When twins are detected at the time of an ultrasound scan preceding a genetic amniocentesis, it is almost always the first time the diagnosis is being made during that pregnancy. The patient is, therefore, inevitably surprised and excited as well as possibly overwhelmed, anxious, or delighted. Two important pieces of information must be given to the patient, and she needs time and some tranquility to consider them. For these reasons, we never proceed with the amniocentesis at this point. The patient is taken off the table and brought into the office where she is asked to consider the following:

1   Since two-thirds of twins in the United States are dizygotic, and this fraction is higher in women aged 35 to 39 years, it is necessary to tap both sacs in order to obtain information on two fetuses which may well be genetically dissimilar. This, of course, involves at least two and possibly more needle insertions, which increases the risk of the procedure.

2   The possibility exists that one twin will be genetically normal while the other is found to have a significant abnormality. The patient and her husband should consider how they might respond to the knowledge that this were the case. Would they abort a normal twin to avoid having an affected child, or would they continue the pregnancy in order to spare that normal fetus. Some people prefer not to have to face this difficult decision and decide to forego amniocentesis altogether. The possibility of aborting only the affected fetus will not be discussed because, although it has been done, it raises moral, technical, and medical issues which are extraordinarily complex and beyond the scope of this text. Practically speaking, this option is simply not available to the overwhelming majority of our patients.

The patient is given another appointment for several days later and sent home to consider these issues. If she elects to keep her new appointment, amniocentesis is performed in the following manner:

Careful scanning is performed until the lies and relative orientation of both twins have been established. Real-

Figure 8

Membranes (*arrow*) can clearly be seen separating the sacs of this twin gestation. *P*, placenta.

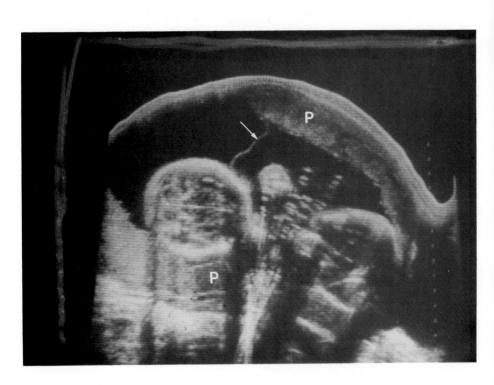

time scanners are ideal for this purpose as their long transducer heads can easily be aligned with each fetal long axis to rapidly and accurately establish the position of both twins. It is almost always possible to see a membrane separating the two fetal sacs (Figure 8). A site is then chosen where the fluid seems to be clearly associated with the sac of the first twin to be tapped. After insertion of the needle and aspiration of a fluid sample, 0.2 to 0.5 cc of indigo carmine, a blue dye, is injected. The needle is then withdrawn, and the patient is quickly scanned again to reassess the fetal positions. Based on the position of the membranes, a second insertion site is selected and the needle is brought as close as possible to the body of the second twin. Fluid is then aspirated; if it is clear, the second sac has been successfully entered. If the fluid is blue-tinged, the first sac has been re-entered and the patient must be rescanned for selection of a third insertion site.

It is important not to use a red dye to avoid confusion with a bloody tap. A case of fetal hyperbilirubinemia secondary to the use of methylene blue as a marker for amniotic fluid has been reported (9). To our knowledge

Evans blue or indigo carmine have not been associated with any adverse fetal effects. The same technique described above can also be used for triplets without using other colored dyes. When, in that instance, clear fluid is aspirated from the second sac, 0.2 to 0.5 cc of indigo carmine should be introduced before withdrawing the needle. If the third tap produces clear fluid, the third sac has been successfully entered. On the other hand, blue-tinged fluid indicates that another attempt is necessary regardless of which of the first two sacs has been re-entered.

In one series of genetic amniocentesis, sampling from both sacs was requested by 20 women with twin gestations (13). In all cases both fetuses were ultrasonically shown to be viable and of normal size. Fluid was successfully obtained from both amniotic sacs in 19 of these 20 cases using the technique described above.

Complications

Two large North American studies have shown no statistically significant increase in the incidence of fetal loss, or complications of pregnancy or delivery when patients receiving second trimester taps were compared to matched controls (31, 37). Both of these studies were published in 1976. One was a nine-center collaborative investigation done in the United States in which 1040 patients who had a total of 1195 taps were compared with 992 controls. The incidence of pregnancy wastage in the week immediately following the amniocentesis was four in 1040, or 0.4%. Based on these data most centers in the United States currently quote a risk of about one in 200 (0.5%) for pregnancy loss associated with a second trimester tap. Considerable expertise has been developed since the American collaborative report was published, and in busy centers the actual incidence of pregnancy wastage today is probably lower than the figure quoted. Since 1978 the total number of pregnancies spontaneously lost within 4 weeks of a second trimester tap at Yale-New Haven Hospital is five in 1683, or 0.3%. At McGill the figures for the same period are 14 in 1684 which results in a corrected incidence of 0.65% when two cases of incompetent cervix and one meningomyelocele are removed from the analysis.

The American study, as well as a large Canadian study, found that the incidence of fetal loss increased with the use of needles of 19 gauge or larger and when more than two insertions were necessary to obtain the fluid. The Canadian study suggested that the pregnancy wastage with more than two insertions during a single amniocentesis was greater than that following a second or even a third tap later in the same pregnancy.

A British study was published in 1978 in which 2428 women undergoing amniocentesis in the first 20 weeks of pregnancy were compared with the same number of matched controls (26). In this investigation an increased fetal loss of 1 to 1.5%, and a "possible increase" of 1 to 1.5% in unexplained abnormalities were observed in the amniocentesis group. So far, these findings have not been duplicated. Speculation about the cause of these disturbing results has included concern about the suitability of the control population, as well as incorporation into the study a group of patients who were referred because of high serum AFP's. In any case, the validity of the British findings remains to be established. Until this is done the extensive North American experience should probably continue to be the basis on which our patients are counseled.

The use of ultrasound

Is it necessary to perform an ultrasound examination prior to a second trimester amniocentesis? This is a legitimate question to ask, even in a textbook of obstetrical ultrasonography. In our opinion, despite some confusion in the literature, the answer is unequivocally affirmative. The American collaborative study did not demonstrate any reduction in maternal complications or fetal loss when ultrasound was used to localize the placenta (31). It should be noted, however, that these data were collected between 1971 and 1973 when the quality of the ultrasound was greatly inferior to that which is now available. The authors of the report were aware of this fact and recommend that the data regarding ultrasound in their study be interpreted with caution. Four sets of twins were scanned for placental localization in that series, and in only one of those cases was the multiple gestation detected.

The Canadian investigators found that a higher percentage of taps were successful and that fluid was more often obtained after one insertion when amniocentesis was preceded by a scan (37). They could not demonstrate, however, that the use of ultrasound affected the incidence of fetal loss or maternal complications.

In several later series (7, 10, 22, 30) the use of ultrasound immediately prior to amniocentesis was shown to be associated with significant reductions in the incidence of bloody taps when compared to procedures done without ultrasound assistance. Karp et al. (20) did not find that the use of ultrasound reduced the number of bloody taps, but Gottesfeld (17) has pointed out that in their series the tap was "usually performed within an hour of the scan." His letter to the editor reiterates the fact that changes in placental and fetal position occur when patients void, move about on the examining table, or have taps performed at times other than during the initial ultrasound examination.

Levine et al. (27) reported on 150 patients divided alternately into one group receiving a scan immediately prior to a tap and another where the tap was performed without ultrasound assistance. These authors could demonstrate no significant reduction in the failure rate (4% vs. 5.3%), incidence of multiple needle insertions (15.3% vs. 15.5%), or proportion of AF samples containing blood (10% vs. 6%) when taps with scans were compared with those without scans. It is interesting, however, that in a report of 3000 cases of second trimester amniocenteses authored by one of the contributors to the paper by Levine et al., ultrasonography was used prior to all the taps in the second half of the series (14). In the last 1000 cases of that series, fluid was obtained on the first attempt in 99.3% of the cases. The authors claim that their improvement over earlier statistics in the series was due to moving the date of tapping from 15 up to 16 weeks from LMP, the recognition of missed abortions at the time of the scan (12 in 1000), and the recognition of misdated pregnancies with subsequent postponement to a more suitable time for the amniocentesis. The latter two explanations, of course, are dependent on data derived from their scans.

Hohler and colleagues (19) found that there was no statistical difference in the incidence of bloody taps whether the placenta was demonstrated to be anterior or posterior immediately prior to the tap. These authors concluded that placental penetration during amniocentesis is not "the major or only cause of bloody taps." Nevertheless, they did advocate scanning prior to the tap in order to accurately locate the placenta; assess fetal position, number, and movement; choose a tap site; and estimate needle penetration depth to reach a pocket of fluid. In their series of 135 patients, the following unsuspected findings were detected by ultrasound examination: two cases of blighted ovum, one fetal death in utero, one set of twins, and six patients who were more than 3 weeks off in calculation of gestational age.

Mennuti et al. (29) studied 333 patients with serum AFP's in the normal range prior to second trimester taps using ultrasound. Using a post-tap elevation in AFP of more than 35% as an indicator of significant feto-maternal bleeding, they divided the patients into two groups. The rate of spontaneous abortion in the group with no significant change in maternal serum AFP was 0.98% (3 in 305) as compared with 14.3% (4 in 28) in the other group. The frequency of patients with predominantly anterior placentas who had significant elevations in post-tap AFP was 15.8% vs. 2.6% to 5.4% for various other placental anatomical locations. Based on these data the authors feel that pregnancy wastage is significantly increased when an anterior placenta is traversed and recommend ultrasonic placental location prior to a tap to more precisely estimate the risk of the procedure when counseling patients. In our experience, however, it is necessary to penetrate an anterior placenta in approximately 20% of cases. Our pregnancy wastage, as cited earlier, is extremely low, and we have not been impressed with an increase in problems with women having anterior placentas. We suggest that until larger series substantiate the findings of Mennuti et al. the risk to patients whose placentas must be traversed in order to obtain fluid be considered minimally increased, if at all.

In summary, the following arguments can be made for the use of ultrasound immediately prior to tapping:

1 It permits diagnosis of multiple gestations, fetal deaths in utero, and missed abortions.
2 It permits misdated pregnancies to be recognized and, if appropriate, the amniocentesis rescheduled.
3 In most hands it reduces the incidence of bloody taps and increases the success rate of the initial insertion.
4 It permits the diagnosis of unsuspected pelvic pathology (e.g., fibroids and ovarian cysts) and gross fetal anomalies (e.g., anencephaly).
5 It turns a blind procedure into one in which the location of the placenta and fetus are known very shortly before the needle insertion.

The last reason listed is certainly not the least important. How many of us would be happy about performing any other kind of surgical procedure with our eyes closed? By way of dramatic illustration of this point, Figure 9 is a midline sagittal scan of a patient at 16 weeks prior to amniocentesis. If, as is usually the case, arbitrary needle insertion were made midway between the symphysis and the top of the fundus, it would go through the thickest part of the placenta directly into the fetus in this instance.

Figure 9

Midline sagittal scan of a fetus at 16 weeks. Blind amniocentesis midway between the top of the uterine fundus and the pubic symphysis would result in traversing the thickest part of the placenta and entering the fetal body in this patient.

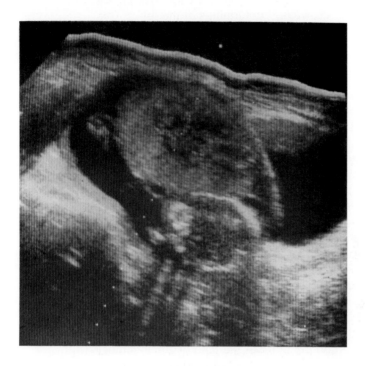

Management following second trimester amniocentesis

As many as 5% of women may pass small quantities of blood and/or fluid vaginally within 48 hrs. of the tap. This represents the retromembranous dissection of fluid from the site of the needle insertion and, if it is self-limited, has no adverse prognostic implications. A very small number of women, however, will continue to leak fluid vaginally for the remainder of their pregnancy. Two potential problems exist for these patients. The first is the possibility of acquiring an ascending infection from the vagina. This is quite unlikely since the tap site is usually not close to the internal cervical os. Nevertheless, these patients should refrain from coitus, douching, and the use of tampons while the leaking persists. For 3 to 4 days following the onset of continuous leakage, temperatures every 6 hrs. and daily white blood cells should be obtained to rule out amnionitis associated with the procedure itself. Following this, normal activities, with the above prohibitions, may be permitted. Any subsequent fever, episode of abdominal pain, or foul vaginal discharge should, of course, be rapidly and thoroughly investigated.

The second potential problem associated with the chronic passage of fluid is severe oligohydramnios with resultant "crowding" deformities of the fetus. This should be looked for with serial scans, but in our experience it is very uncommon following amniocentesis with a 20- or 22-gauge needle. Absence of marked oligohydramnios in association with chronic leakage reflects the rapid turnover of amniotic fluid within the gestational sac and the large quantities of this fluid which are constantly being produced.

Grossly bloody taps which do not clear may be associated with fetal exsanguination if a large fetal vessel has been lacerated (39). Unfortunately, there is currently nothing that can be done to correct this problem in the second trimester, and so electronic fetal heart rate monitoring is not useful after a bloody tap. If a Kleihauer-Betke stain subsequently indicates that a significant quantity of fetal blood has contaminated the tap, the patient can be recalled in 24 hrs. to verify that the fetus is still alive.

Isolated case reports have described serious sequelae of fetal organ puncture at the time of amniocentesis (3, 8, 11, 12, 15, 25, 29, 35). The relative sparcity of these reports and the absence of fetal injury attributable to needle puncture in several large series suggest that this is not a very common occurrence. The fetus seems to move away from the needle if it is touched during the procedure, although small skin dimples have been reported in 1 to 4% of cases in some series (6). The quantity of fluid relative to the size of a second trimester fetus makes it unlikely that a needle would do more than nick the skin unless it were thrust into the uterus with excessive force or the fetus were trapped in an area where it could not move. Ultrasound scanning immediately prior to the tap certainly should reduce the incidence of fetal puncture, but this has not yet been conclusively demonstrated.

Third trimester amniocentesis

While the technique of obtaining fluid is essentially the same, there are important differences between taps done in the second trimester. As mentioned at the beginning of this chapter, third trimester taps are done for a variety of reasons but most frequently to assess fetal lung maturity before elective or premature delivery. It is sometimes necessary to do more than one amniocentesis during the same pregnancy when, for example, an immature L/S ratio has been obtained on the initial tap, or an Rh-sensitized patient requires serial

$\triangle OD_{450}$ analysis. The amniocentesis may be more difficult technically than second trimester taps in obese patients with anterior placentas as well as in those with oligohydramnios. Finally, a larger fetus in relatively less fluid is more susceptible to trauma with the needle.

When ultrasound was not available, physicians would pick one of three general areas to tap:

1 over the fetal small parts
2 in the nuchal area
3 just above the symphysis.

Since there is generally between 800 and 1200 cc of amniotic fluid in late pregnancy, fluid can usually be found with "blind" insertion of a needle into one of the above areas. However, with this approach the positions of the placenta and cord are unknown. While fluid can usually be obtained from the vicinity of the fetal limbs, this may be where an anterior placenta is thickest. Also, if the nuchal area is chosen and the umbilical cord is around the neck of the fetus, it is immobile and consequently more likely to be punctured by a needle than if it were floating freely. For these reasons we strongly feel that ultrasound scanning prior to a third trimester tap is as essential as that preceding an amniocentesis in the second trimester.

Method

The selection of a needle insertion site at the time of the scan should be through a placenta-free window whenever possible. If placental penetration is unavoidable, then it should not be near the cord insertion. Obviously, one should try to find a site that is as far as possible from the fetal head and other vital organs. In cases of oligohydramnios, small pockets of fluid must be carefully examined to be sure that they do not contain loops of trapped cord (Figure 10). If no accessible accumulation of fluid can be detected ultrasonically and a suprapubic tap is impossible, then the tap should simply not be done. With experience one learns not only where to tap, but when *not* to tap (Figure 11).

In some obese patients, especially if there is an anterior placenta, a pocket of fluid may be located that is beyond the length of a standard 9-cm needle. In these cases the distance from the skin surface to the fluid should be measured with a graticule on the scanner and a 15-cm 20- or 22-gauge needle used. It may also be helpful to perform these scans with a 2.25 MHz transducer in order to obtain greater penetration with the ultrasound beam. With this technique we have been able to obtain fluid samples successfully from women

Figure 10

The tip of the amniocentesis needle can be seen within a small pocket of amniotic fluid on this real-time scan.

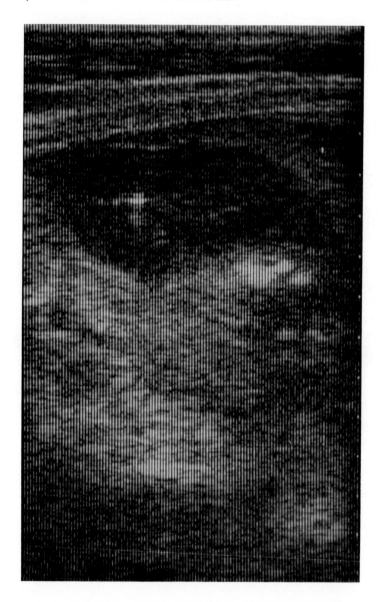

who were so heavy that the size of their uterus could not be determined by abdominal palpation.

Complications

Potential adverse sequelae to a third trimester tap include premature rupture of the membranes, premature labor, amnionitis, trauma to the fetus or cord, and abdominal wall hematoma. Far fewer series of third trimester taps have been reported than those performed in the second trimester. An Australian review of 2003 consecutive amniocenteses on 1704 patients

Figure 11

A small pocket of amniotic fluid containing several loops of cord. This pocket should *not* be tapped.

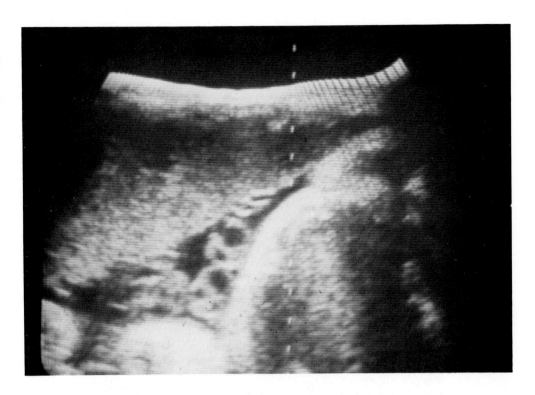

in late pregnancy was published in 1979 (32). In this series all the patients were scanned immediately prior to the procedure and then tapped with a 22-gauge lumbar puncture needle. In 790 patients the amniocentesis was performed through an anterior placenta. All Rh-negative women who had a tap performed through an anterior placenta were given anti-D gammaglobulin. Suprapubic amniocenteses were performed in 10 patients in whom a bulky placenta covered most of the anterior uterine wall, and normal volumes of fluid were present in association with a high fetal head. Less than 2 cc of AF were obtained on 26 occasions (1.3%). One hundred twenty-six (6.3%) of the specimens were grossly blood-stained, and 89% of these were obtained by transplacental puncture. In one of these cases the fluid was later seen to be heavily blood-stained when labor was induced 3 days after the tap. The delivery was uncomplicated, but the cord hemoglobin was 12 g/100 ml and a 2-cm subchorionic clot was noted on the placenta. No fetal morbidity was demonstrated in the other 125 patients with bloody taps. None of the patients in this series was rhesus-sensitized and there was no evidence of fetal laceration or stab wounds. There were no fetal deaths. Labor commenced within 24 hrs. in 42 patients (2.1%).

Platt et al. (33) utilized real-time ultrasound immediately prior to 14 second trimester and 136 third trimester taps in 143 patients. In 146 procedures (including five patients with premature rupture of membranes), fluid was obtained following a single needle insertion. There were no cases of amnionitis, premature rupture of membranes within 48 hrs., or fetal trauma. In one case of twins with hydramnios in which both sacs were tapped, premature labor began 10 hrs. after the procedure.

The data from those two series are very encouraging. In experienced hands, third trimester amniocentesis performed immediately after an ultrasound examination has been shown to be a safe and useful procedure. It must be emphasized, however, that other series (38) testify to the potentially serious problems that may result from amniocentesis, and this procedure must always be performed with the respect and care given to an invasive technique.

Management following third trimester amniocentesis

In the third trimester, unlike the second, a fetus is potentially salvageable if amniocentesis jeopardizes its life in utero. One's management following a tap should reflect that difference. If the amniocentesis has been entirely uneventful and clear fluid has been obtained, demonstration of fetal cardiac activity in the normal range by Doppler or real-time ultrasound is sufficient. If, on the other hand, the tap has been bloody or the fetus has been hit by the needle, electronic fetal heart rate monitoring (EFM) should be performed until the operator is satisfied that there is no distress in utero.

Picker et al. (32) noted that in many patients a marked slowing of the fetal heart occurs immediately following amniocentesis in the third trimester. They suggested that this may occur because of maternal supine hypotension and/or stimulation of the umbilical cord when movement of the fetal limbs brushes the cord against the needle. In all their cases when bradycardia was observed the rate recovered spontaneously. Two situations can be envisioned, however, in which EFM could reflect more ominous conditions. If a large fetal vessel is lacerated by the needle, significant blood loss may occur, resulting in accelerating tachycardia associated with a loss of variability and then perhaps the development of a prolonged bradycardia, spontaneous decelerations, or a sinusoidal pattern. Alternatively, if a hematoma in the cord were produced by trauma at the time of the amniocentesis, one would expect to see a profound and prolonged bradycardia. The only therapy for a major fetal bleed or cord occlusion is rapid delivery by emergency cesarean section. For this reason we strongly advocate performing all third trimester taps in the hospital where EFM equipment and rapid access to an operating room are available.

If a tap produces bloody fluid which does not clear and electronic fetal heart rate monitoring is within normal limits for 1 hr. after the tap, the patient may go home, but a sample of the fluid should be sent for a Kleihauer-Betke stain. Should the report of this test indicate a significant fetal bleed, the patient should have a non-stress test the following day.

Rh-negative patients

There is no question that Rh-negative women may become sensitized following amniocentesis in either the second or third trimester (34). In some centers after each amniocentesis Rh immune globulin (Rh IG) is administered to all Rh-negative women having Rh-positive consorts. In other institutions Rh IG is not administered to these patients if the placenta is posterior and the tap is macroscopically bloodless. Since the precise margins of the placenta are often not known, however, the latter approach may not be free of failures.

How much Rh IG should be administered following amniocentesis? The answer to this question is currently unclear. A full 300-μg dose should cover the introduction of 30 cc of Rh-positive whole blood into the maternal circulation. A 50-μg dose, which should cover a 5-cc bleed, has been marketed for administration to patients following first trimester abortions. Many centers administer this "mini-dose" following second trimester taps. However, in Mennuti et al.'s study of post-second trimester tap maternal serum AFP elevations, one fetus was identified that had an estimated feto-maternal bleed of more than 10 cc (29). This suggests that a routinely administered dose of 150 μg might be more appropriate than the marketed mini-dose preparation. An alternative approach would be to perform a quantitative Kleihauer-Betke count and tailor the amount of Rh IG given to the estimated feto-maternal bleed. In the third trimester, a full 300-μg dose should be given unless quantitative assessment suggests that for a particular patient a smaller amount will be sufficient.

Intrauterine transfusion

The widespread use of Rh immune globulin has dramatically decreased the incidence of Rh hemolytic disease. Nevertheless, a small but steady number of severely sensitized women continue to require sophisticated perinatal care. For these patients transfusion in utero may offer the best chance for fetal survival.

Liley's original description of an intrauterine transfusion (IUT) in 1963 involved the introduction of radiopaque material into the amniotic fluid by amniocentesis (28). Opacification of the fetal gastrointestinal tract with swallowed contrast material was later observed on anteroposterior and cross table lateral films. Using maternal skin markers as reference points, an entry site into the fetal peritoneal cavity was then selected. If the fetus required manipulation to convert its position to one more suitable for transfusion, additional sets of radiographs were required prior to performing the IUT. After inserting a 16-gauge Touhy needle into the fetal abdominal cavity, a catheter was threaded through it and the needle removed. Proper catheter placement was verified by injecting a small amount of radiopaque material and taking another x-ray. A characteristic spread of contrast around bowel or under the diaphragm demonstrated that the catheter lay free within the fetal abdominal cavity, and the transfusion was then performed. If the catheter was not correctly placed, a second needle was inserted, more contrast was injected, and another radiograph was taken. This procedure was repeated until proper placement was verified.

Numerous modifications of this technique, including the use of image intensification fluoroscopy, have been attempted to improve its safety and ease of performance. An important concern regarding any approach which relies on x-ray localization of the targeted peritoneal cavity, however, is unavoidable fetal radiation exposure that may increase the risk of leukemia and childhood malignancies. The amount of radiation delivered to a fetus being transfused in utero may not be trivial, especially when one considers that multiple procedures are often necessary.

In an attempt to diminish fetal radiation exposure, ultrasound has been used to diagnose hydrops, identify the fetal lie, localize the placental position, select an insertion site, and follow the progress of the needle as it is passed into the fetal abdomen. After a report in 1976 (18) describing the selection of an insertion site with ultrasound and introduction of the transfusion needle through a needle aspiration transducer, several techniques of performing IUT's with ultrasonic assistance have been published (1).

A detailed discussion of the timing of transfusion, volume of blood to be introduced, rate of blood transfusion, fetal heart rate monitoring in transfused fetuses, and timing of delivery is beyond the scope of this chapter. The interested reader is referred to a review of these issues (1).

The following description of the technique used to perform IUT's at Yale-New Haven Hospital is taken from a recent report of the experience with this method over a 3 1/2-year period:

At Yale-New Haven Hospital all IUT's are performed in the obstetrical ultrasound room. The patient lies on a mat that covers a wooden x-ray cassette frame. Before transfusion 5 to 10 mg of diazepam are given intravenously to decrease fetal movement, and the patient is scanned with both static and real-time equipment. Hydrops can be diagnosed at this time by demonstrating fetal ascites, edema of the skin over the skull or abdomen, and placental hypertrophy. The fetus can also be manipulated until it lies in a position that is satisfactory for transfusion. This can be accomplished, in some cases, by rolling the fetus laterally or by having the patient assume a kneeling knee-chest position for a few minutes prior to re-examination in a supine position. Sometimes, however, it is necessary to perform external version of a fetus in breech presentation to a vertex or vice versa.

After the fetus has been coaxed into a suitable position, careful scanning is performed to locate an entry site into the fetal abdomen below the level of the umbilical vein and above the bladder. Immediately before introducing the needle, the static scanner probe is placed over the site selected for maternal skin insertion and directed along the precise path to be taken by the needle (Figure 12). The depth from the maternal skin surface to mid-fetal abdomen can be directly read from a graticule that appears on the image display. After rapid aseptic and anesthetic preparation of the skin, the needle is decisively advanced into the fetal abdomen. A needle aspiration transducer is not employed. Passage of the needle is followed with real-time observation. Appropriate placement is verified by injecting 3 to 5 ml of Renografin-60 through the needle and taking a single anteroposterior radiograph 15 to 30 sec. after the injection. Alternatively, 1 to 2 cc of air can be injected under real-time observation. If the needle is properly placed, bubbles of air may be noted rising to the superior aspect of the fetal peritoneal cavity.

After successful introduction of the needle, a closed system is created by removing the needle's stylet and connecting intravenous tubing with a three-way stopcock from the container of blood to the needle hub.

Figure 12

This is a transverse scan of the abdomen of a fetus immediately prior
to intrauterine transfusion. The spine is at 9 o'clock, and the graticule
is positioned along the path of needle insertion. The level of this scan
is midway between the entrance of the umbilical vein into the
abdomen and the top of the fetal bladder.

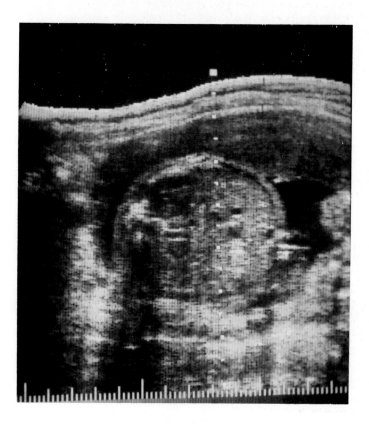

An intraperitoneal catheter is not introduced unless a
significant amount of ascites is present and aspiration
of some of the fluid is anticipated. Blood is manually
injected from a 30-ml syringe attached to the stopcock.
The fetal heart is visually monitored with real-time
ultrasound scanning throughout the procedure, and the
transfused blood can be seen to accumulate within
dependent portions of the fetal peritoneal cavity as the
transfusion proceeds (Figure 13). Injection is performed
at an average rate of 5 to 10 ml/min., and the system
is periodically broken by detaching the tubing from the
needle to look for backflow. The maximum quantity of
blood infused is calculated from the following formula:
(gestation in weeks − 20) × 10 ml (5). This is used
only as a guide, however, as the transfusion may be
stopped prior to administering this quantity of blood if
increased resistance to injection or significant backflow
through the needle is noted. After the transfusion has

Figure 13

A rim of blood in the abdomen of a fetus after intrauterine transfusion.

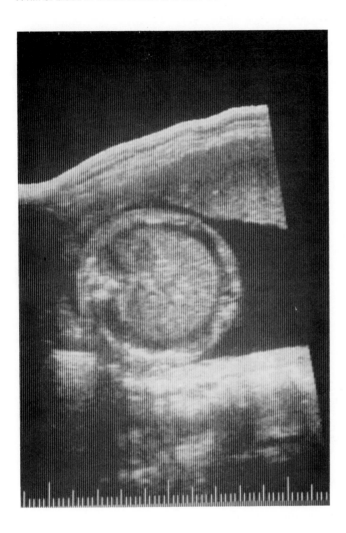

been completed, the stylet is replaced and the needle withdrawn. The fetus is then followed with external fetal heart rate monitoring for a period of at least 1 hr. The patient is discharged the next morning, following real-time documentation of normal cardiac activity.

As of March 1981, the technique described above has been utilized to perform 51 transfusions in 22 severely Rh-sensitized completed pregnancies. The neonatal survival rate was 77%; 57% (four of seven) of the hydropic fetuses and 87% (13 of 15) of those with no antenatal evidence of ascites survived. Thirty-five percent (six of 17) of the neonatal survivors received their initial transfusion at 26.5 weeks or earlier. One fetus in a set of twins was successfully transfused at 29

Figure 14

Instruments used during fetoscopy. *A*, needlescope; *B*, 26-gauge needle used for aspiration of blood; *C*, cannula with Y-piece through which the needle is inserted; *D*, trocar.

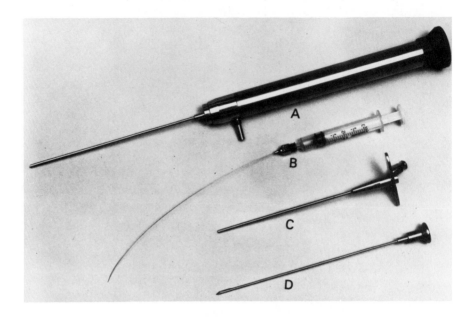

1/2 weeks. Both neonates were found to be Rh-positive, and both survived. The statistics from this series are as good as the best of these from series using x-ray as an aid for needle placement.

Fetoscopy and fetal blood sampling

Although the availability of amniotic fluid has been responsible for enormous progress in prenatal genetic diagnosis, there are limitations to the amount of information the fluid can provide. Of the cells extruded into AF, 90% are dead or dying, and neither they nor the fluid itself reflect all the metabolic functions of the fetus. Therefore, some investigators have developed techniques to directly view the fetus, biopsy its skin, and sample its blood. All these procedures are accomplished through a small endoscope and specially designed cannula for fetal blood drawing.

Fetal blood sampling is the most frequent reason for performing fetoscopy today. A variety of analyses can be performed on fetal blood. Globin chain synthesis studies can be performed on red blood cells to diagnose hemoglobinopathies such as thalassemia major and sickle cell disease. White blood cells can be studied for functional abnormalities such as chronic granulomatous disease. Serum can be assayed for clotting disorders such as hemophilia. Numerous other tests are also possible such as platelet counts and enzyme analyses. The success of these studies, however, depends upon obtaining samples from the fetal circulation that are as uncontaminated with maternal blood and amniotic fluid as possible.

Ultrasound plays an essential role in fetal blood sampling. The best site for obtaining pure fetal blood is from large vessels in the cord root, 1 to 2 cm from its insertion on the placenta. These vessels can be entered with a 26- or 27-gauge needle and samples of blood aspirated under direct vision. Careful scanning prior to beginning the procedure permits identification of the cord insertion site. In addition, a site of entry into the amniotic cavity can be selected which minimizes the chances of injuring the fetus while permitting access to the target vessels.

The instruments used in fetal blood drawing include a 15-cm long non-flexible fiberoptic fetoscope, a cannula with a Y side arm having a diameter of 2.2 by 2.7 mm, and a 26- or 27-gauge sampling needle (Figure 14). After the entry site has been selected and the location of the cord insertion determined, the cannula is introduced into the amniotic sac. The cannula's trochar is then withdrawn and the fetoscope and needle inserted into its central lumen and side arm, respectively. Upon visually locating a vessel in the cord root, the needle is advanced until the vessel is pierced. An assistant then aspirates a sample of blood, an aliquot of which is immediately measured in a Coulter cell sizer. The difference in red cell volume between maternal and fetal cells permits verification of the source of the specimen. The cell sizer allows one to be certain that a sample is fetal in origin and to quantify the degree of maternal contamination in a "mixed specimen."

Fetoscopy has been used to directly view the face, extremities, or genitalia in situations where the fetus is at risk for conditions affecting these structures. The practical utility of this approach, however, is limited by technical difficulties associated with the magnification imposed by small diameter endoscopes. With the improved image quality of newer ultrasound equipment, a great deal of this morphological detail can now be visualized without subjecting the patient to the potential morbidity of an invasive procedure. It should be remembered that in the hands of experienced operators fetoscopy is associated with a related abortion rate of approximately 5%, an incidence of delivery prior to the 36th week of gestation of about

9%, and leakage of significant amounts of amniotic fluid in about 1% of cases.

Therapy in utero

There is no doubt that ultrasound will have a primary role in the exciting developments emerging in the next decade surrounding the treatment of a variety of conditions in utero. Perhaps the most exciting potential for fetoscopy is the ability it provides to inject drugs, enzymes, or clones of cells directly into the fetus through the umbilical cord. Fetuses deficient in a specific enzyme or other essential substance might thereby become salvageable.

Treatment of potentially lethal obstructive conditions such as posterior urethral valves or hydrocephaly is now becoming a reality. Under ultrasonic direction specially designed catheters, which empty into the amniotic fluid, have been inserted into the fetal bladder or cranium and left in utero. These catheters relieve pressure and thereby spare renal and cerebral tissue from the destructive forces of compression caused by the obstructed flow of fluid.

References

1 **Berkowitz, R.L.:** Intrauterine transfusion, 1980: An update. Clin. Perinatol. 7:2, 1980.

2 **Berkowitz, R.L., Hobbins, J.C.:** A reevaluation of the value of hCS determination in the management of prolonged pregnancy. Obstet. Gynecol. 49:156, 1977.

3 **Berner, H.W., Seisler, E.P., Barlow, J.:** Fetal cardiac tamponade, a complication of amniocentesis. Obstet. Gynecol. 40:599, 1972.

4 **Bobitt, J.R., Ledger, W.J.:** Amniotic fluid analysis—its role in maternal and neonatal infection. Obstet. Gynecol. 51:56, 1978.

5 **Bowman, J.M.:** Rh erythroblastosis 1975. Semin. Hematol. 12:189, 1975.

6 **Broome, D.L., Wilson, M.G., Weiss, B., Kellogg, B.:** Needle puncture of fetus: A complication of second-trimester amniocentesis. Am. J. Obstet. Gynecol. 126:2, 247, 1976.

7 **Chandra, P., Nitowsky, H.M., Marion, R., Koenigsberg, M., Taben, E., Kava, H.W.:** Experience with sonography as an adjunct to amniocentesis for prenatal diagnosis of fetal genetic disorders. Am. J. Obstet. Gynecol. 133:519, 1979.

8 **Cook, L.N., Shott, R.J., Andrews, B.F.:** Fetal complications of diagnostic amniocentesis: A review and report of a case with pneumothorax. Pediatrics 53:421, 1974.

9 **Cowett, R.M., Hakanson, D.O., Kocon, R.W., Oh, W.:** Untoward neonatal effect of intraamniotic administration of methylene blue. Obstet. Gynecol. (Suppl.) 48:74, 1976.

10 Crandon, A.J., Peel, K.R.: Amniocentesis with and without ultrasound guidance. Br. J. Obstet. Gynaecol. 86:1, 1979.

11 Cross, H.E., Maumenee, A.E.: Letter to the editor: Ocular trauma during amniocentesis. N. Engl. J. Med. 287:993, 1972.

12 Egley, C.C.: Laceration of fetal spleen during amniocentesis. Am. J. Obstet. Gynecol. 116:582, 1973.

13 Elias, S., Gerbie, A.B., Simpson, J.L., Nadler, H.L., Sabbagha, R.E., Shkolnik, A.: Genetic amniocentesis in twin gestations. Am. J. Obstet. Gynecol. 138:169, 1980.

14 Golbus, M.S., Loughman, W.D., Epstein, C.J., Halbasch, G., Stephens, J.D., Hall, B.D.: Prenatal genetic diagnosis in 3000 amniocenteses. N. Engl. J. Med. 300:157, 1979.

15 Gottdiener, J.S., Ellison, R.C., Lorenzo, R.L.: Arteriovenous fistula after fetal penetration at amniocentesis. N. Engl. J. Med. 293:1302, 1975.

16 Gottesfeld, K.R.: Ultrasound in obstetrics. Clin. Obstet. Gynecol. 21:311, 1978.

17 Gottesfeld, K.R.: Midtrimester amniocentesis: Letter to the editor. Obstet. Gynecol. 53:534, 1979.

18 Hobbins, J.C., Davis, C.D., Webster, J.: A new technique utilizing ultrasound to aid in intrauterine transfusion. J. Clin. Ultrasound 4:135, 1976.

19 Hohler, C.W., Doherty, R.A., Lea, J., Newhouse, J., Felix, J.: Ultrasound placental site in relation to bloody taps in midtrimester amniocentesis. Obstet. Gynecol. 52:555, 1978.

20 Karp, L.E., Rothwell, R., Conrad, S.H., Hoehn, H.W., Hickok, D.E.: Ultrasonic placental localization and bloody taps in midtrimester amniocentesis for prenatal genetic diagnosis. Obstet. Gynecol. 50:589, 1977.

21 Karp, L.E., Schiller, H.S.: Meconium staining of amniotic fluid at midtrimester amniocentesis. Obstet. Gynecol. 50:47s, 1977.

22 Kerenyi, T.D., Walker, B.: The preventability of "bloody taps" in second trimester amniocentesis by ultrasound scanning. Obstet. Gynecol. 50:61, 1977.

23 King, C.R., Prescott, G., Pernoll, M.: Significance of meconium in midtrimester diagnostic amniocentesis. Am. J. Obstet. Gynecol. 132:667, 1978.

24 Knox, G.E., Huddleston, J.F., Flowers, C.E., Management of prolonged pregnancy: Results of a prospective randomized trial. Am. J. Obstet. Gynecol. 134:376, 1979.

25 Lamb, M.P.: Gangrene of a fetal limb due to amniocentesis. Br. J. Obstet. Gynaecol. 82:829, 1975.

26 Leoffler, F.E., ed.: An assessment of the hazards of amniocentesis. Br. J. Obstet. Gynaecol. (Suppl. 2) 85: 1978.

27 Levine, S.C., Filly, R.A., Golbus, M.S.: Ultrasonography for guidance of amniocentesis in genetic counseling. Clin. Genet. 14:133, 1978.

28 Liley, A.W.: Liquor amnii analysis in the management of the pregnancy

complicated by rhesus sensitization. Am. J. Obstet. Gynecol. 82:1359, 1961.

29 **Mennuti, M.T., Brummond, W., Crombleholme, W.R., Schwarz, R.H., Arvan, D.A.:** Fetal-maternal bleeding associated with genetic amniocentesis. Obstet. Gynecol. 55:48, 1980.

30 **Nelson, L.H., Goodman, H.O., Brown, S.H.:** Ultrasonography preceding diagnostic amniocentesis and its effect on amniotic fluid cell growth. Obstet. Gynecol. 50:65, 1977.

31 **NICHD National Registry for Amniocentesis Study Group:** Midtrimester amniocentesis for prenatal diagnosis. J.A.M.A. 236:13, 1471, 1976.

32 **Picker, R.H., Smith, D.H., Saunders, D.M., Pennington, J.C.:** A review of 2,003 consecutive amniocenteses performed under ultrasonic control in late pregnancy. Aust. N. Z. J. Obstet. Gynaecol. 13:83, 1979.

33 **Platt, L.D., Manning, F.A., Lemay, M.:** Realtime B-scan-directed amniocentesis. Am. J. Obstet. Gynecol. 130:700, 1978.

34 **Queenan, J.R.:** *Modern Management of the Rh Problem*, 2nd ed. Harper and Row, Hagerstown, Md., 1977, pp. 64–70.

35 **Reckwood, A.M.K.:** A case of ileal atresia and ileocutaneous fistula caused by amniocentesis. J. Pediatr. 91:312, 1977.

36 **Sandler, M.A., Sznewajs, S.M., Bityk, L.L.:** The effect of the distended urinary bladder on placental position and its importance in amniocentesis. Radiology 130:195, 1979.

37 **Simpson, N.E., Dallaire, L., Miller, J.R., Siminovich, L., Hamerton, J.L., Miller, J., McKeen, C.:** Prenatal diagnosis of genetic disease in Canada: Report of a collaborative study. Can. Med. Assoc. J. 115:739, 1976.

38 **Young, B.K.:** Report on third trimester amniocentesis at Bellevue Hospital of New York University Medical Center, N.Y., N.Y. In *Antenatal Diagnosis*, NIH Publication No. 79-1973, April 1979, p. II-65.

39 **Young, P.E., Matson, M.R., Jones, O.W.:** Fetal exsanguination and other vascular injuries from midtrimester genetic amniocentesis. Am. J. Obstet. Gynecol. 129:21, 1977.

Ultrasound Evaluation of Fetal Dynamics

Introduction

Pediatricians are trained to relate an infant's behavior to its condition. One of the first clues that a child is sick is that it becomes lethargic, and neurological assessment of an infant relates, in part, to its reaction to stimuli. Therefore, it was a logical extrapolation for investigators to attempt to correlate fetal behavior with fetal condition, once real-time ultrasound allowed direct observation of the fetus.

Fetal breathing

Prior to the advent of real-time ultrasound, fetal physiologists were able to demonstrate in animals that fetuses regularly produced thoracic excursions that were indistinguishable from breathing motions made by neonates. Oxford investigators found that the fetal lamb exhibited breathing motions about 80% of the time, and that it was possible to experimentally affect this phenomenon (1, 9). They observed, for instance, that breathing motions stopped when the lamb's pO_2 was lowered or when it was subjected to tranquilizers and narcotics (2). Breathing could be stimulated by glucose and by raising the lamb's pCO_2. Manning et al. (7) demonstrated that the fetal lamb would abruptly cease breathing efforts when its mother inhaled cigarette smoke or was injected with nicotine. Since nicotine injected directly into the fetal lamb caused no such response, it was surmised that the fetal apnea resulted from relative hypoxia caused by the drug's effect on uterine blood flow. Fox et al. (3) later demonstrated that fetal breathing virtually ceased after maternal consumption of 1 oz. of 80-proof alcohol.

The Oxford group reported the presence of human fetal breathing with M-mode ultrasound techniques. Their findings were very similar to those in fetal lambs with regard to time spent breathing and the conditions under which there was a decrease in breathing activity.

But methodological questions were raised regarding the adequacy of amplitude information without

Figure 1

Real-time longitudinal scan of fetus showing diaphragm (arrows). *L*, lung.

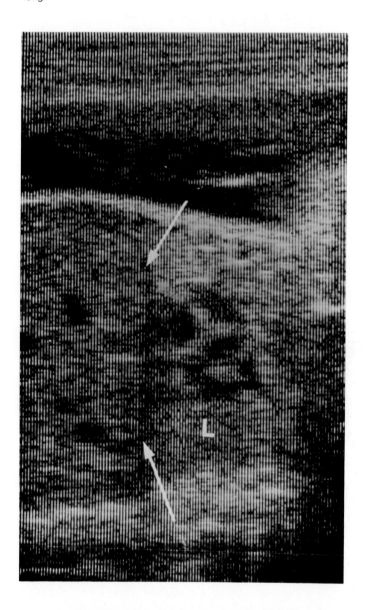

anatomical reference. In the past several years the linear array has become a popular tool for observing the typical diaphragmatic movements made during fetal breathing and measuring this activity, rather than attempting to interpret interrupted chicken scratches on a strip chart recorder. Most investigators have chosen to study fetal breathing with longitudinal scans (Figure 1). During inspiration the anterior chest wall moves inward by about 2 to 5 mm; and the abdominal wall moves outward by 3 to 8 mm. The excursions involved in this paradoxical movement of chest and abdomen are large enough to be visually perceived on real-time.

Many beautifully designed studies have been carried out with real-time to observe normal variations in fetal breathing patterns and to correlate various pathological conditions with fetal breathing responses. Patrick et al. (8) demonstrated that fetuses studied for 24 continuous hrs. spend an average of 31% of their time breathing and that predictable time-dependent variations could be demonstrated. The peaks were at 2 to 3 hr. postprandial and between 4:00 and 7:00 in the morning. Normal fetuses could have apneic periods lasting as long as 120 min. The breathing rate was found to be significantly faster in premature fetuses compared with those at term. Breath-to-breath intervals were generally 0.5 to 1.0 sec. in the 30-week fetus compared with an interval of 1.0 to 1.5 sec. in the 38- to 39-week fetus. Some investigators disagree as to whether regular fetal breathing occurs during quiet sleep. Most agree, however, that the typical irregular pattern of fetal breathing generally is present when the fetus is in active rapid eye movement (REM) sleep, a state in which it spends about 60% of its time at term.

There is strong evidence that the human fetus ceases breathing movements when it is hypoxic. Commonly used electronic fetal monitoring (EFM) tests to assess the condition are very sensitive in predicting a normal fetus but are notorious for their inability to specifically identify one that is compromised. Manning et al. (6) attempted to see if the addition of a fetal breathing test would enhance the specificity of either the non-stress test (NST) or contraction stress test (CST). The end point of the fetal breathing test was very simple: The test was positive if the fetus demonstrated any breathing activity during a 20-min. observation period and negative if it did not. The investigators found that fetuses confirmed to be compromised by evidence of intrapartum asphyxia with EFM monitoring, or low APGAR scores, virtually never made breathing motions. Not all apneic fetuses were shown to be compromised, however, and the false-positive rate for fetal apnea alone was high. If, on the other hand, fetal breathing was absent *and* the NST was non-reactive, the fetus had a greater chance of being compromised than if either test was positive by itself. Similar results were found when the fetal breathing test was combined with the CST (4). In effect, the addition of the fetal breathing test appeared to decrease the false-positive rate of the CST or NST.

Although some studies have tried to correlate abnormal breathing patterns with various abnormal conditions, they have been inconclusive. These studies suffer from an inability to easily document viewer observations on some form of hard copy. The alternative of counting breathing motions on real-time is an extremely tedious, and, therefore, impractical exercise.

Early investigation in the fetal lamb demonstrated that an experimentally asphyxiated animal would intersperse periods of apnea with large gasping-like thoracic excursions just before demise. This finding in the laboratory animal has been used to explain why the asphyxiated human fetus aspirates meconium, but to our knowledge human fetal gasping has not been seen with real-time. Hiccoughs are often seen in completely normal fetuses, however, and should not be confused with fetal gasping.

We feel that the clinical use of real-time analysis of fetal breathing is questionable until more investigation demonstrates that quantification of this activity is worth the considerable effort necessary for its accomplishment. However, there does seem to be enough evidence to suggest that observation of the presence or absence of fetal breathing is useful when used in conjunction with other tests of fetal condition. Even though ideally one would like to evaluate a fetus for 30-min. periods, if one demonstrates breathing activity anytime during this ultrasonic "window," the test can probably be discontinued. It is unclear whether an arbitrary limit of 20 or 30 min. is a fair test of fetal well-being, but prolongation beyond this time span becomes impractical.

Investigation is in progress to correlate glucose-stimulated respirations with fetal condition. Although this technique may decrease the amount of false-positive tests, there are insufficient data yet to determine if a glucose load will coax respirations from a compromised fetus and thereby result in a higher incidence of false-negative tests.

Fetal activity

When an intrauterine demise has occurred, women will either report that their fetus gradually became less active prior to cessation of perceived fetal movement or, less frequently, that there was a sudden flurry of activity followed by a complete absence of movement.

Sadovsky and Yaffe (13), recognizing that fetal movements represented a valuable indicator of fetal condition, initiated a program of screening through quantification of maternally perceived fetal movement. He used the daily fetal movement recording (DFMR), which is the total number of movements perceived by the mother over a 24-hr. period. It is obtained by counting movements for 30 min. three times a day. If fewer than three movements for 30 min. per hour are detected, the woman continues counting for a period of 6 to 12 hrs. The DFMR was found to vary considerably in normal pregnancies and to sometimes fluctuate dramatically for individual patients. Therefore, Sadovsky and Polishuk (12) concluded that there was no significance to the absolute number of movements recorded, provided that they did not cease entirely during a period of 12 hrs. When there was a reduction in fetal movements up to their cessation for at least 12 hrs. and fetal heartbeats were still audible, this was referred to as the "movements alarm signal" (MAS). In 22 of 50 cases who had the MAS, death occurred in utero. The other 28 fetuses were delivered alive as soon as this signal was detected, and 24 of these neonates survived. The authors concluded that the MAS is indicative of severe distress in utero and impending fetal death.

Since real-time ultrasound allows direct visualization of fetal movement, this modality has been used to quantify fetal movements more precisely. However, the transducer can capture only a portion of the third trimester fetus at one time, and, therefore, visualization of all fetal movements is difficult. Roberts et al. (10) attempted to bypass this problem by concentrating on fetal trunk movements (FTM's) on a transverse scan. Total fetal activity (TFA) was defined as the amount of time the fetus spent either breathing or moving and was expressed as a percentage of the total observation time. When monitoring 21 normal patients for 1 hr. per 3-hr. period over 24 hrs., a marked circadian rhythm in FTM for all patients was noted. The incidence of FTM was found to be fairly constant during the day but greatest in late evening and in the early hours of the morning. These authors also found that, although the incidence of fetal movement in the third trimester did not vary with gestational age, movements of fetuses between 28 and 34 weeks were generally of shorter duration than those of later gestation. Despite the fact that the mean incidences of FTM and fetal respiratory movements (FRM) during the day were 16% and 37%, respectively, there was a large range in incidence of both of these variables at any particular hour of the day. While it was, therefore, not uncommon to find a very low incidence of fetal respiration or, alternatively, fetal movements, in a 30-min. recording period, it was rare to find a TFA of less than 10% in any 1/2-hr. period or absence of either activity over a period of 10 min.

This group has studied 25 pregnancies complicated by diabetes mellitus (11). In 15 well-controlled insulin-dependent diabetic women with uncomplicated pregnancies, the FRM and TFA were significantly higher than in non-diabetics, but FTM's were the same. In six pregnancies with obstetrical complications, however, TFA levels below 10% correlated well with abnormal NST's or fetal distress in labor.

Manning et al. (5) have designed a score composed of five biophysical variables: fetal breathing, fetal movements, observed fetal tone, quantitative amniotic fluid volume, and the non-stress test. Similar to the famous APGAR score, each parameter was given a value of 0 when abnormal and 2 when normal. A perfect score, therefore, was 10. This method of fetal evelution was used in 216 high risk pregnancies. Although the false-negative rate was very low for any of the five variables used independently, the false-positive rate was quite high for each (over 50%). A combination of the above tests enhanced the predictive value. If all variables were normal, the perinatal mortality rate (PNM) was 0. When, on the other hand, all of the variables were abnormal, the PNM was 60%.

This type of scoring system, while being comprehensive, incorporates a number of indirectly related variables together and suffers somewhat by reducing the richness of data to a single number. Nevertheless, the concept of systematically approaching the fetus with regard to its various basic activities is very appealing.

Many more years of study will be required before it can be firmly established that real-time assessment of basic fetal functions is clinically worth the considerable effort necessary to quantify these activities. Investigation of fetal activity, however, has already provided some extremely important information about fetal behavior.

References

1 **Boddy, K., Dawes, G.S., Fisher, R., Pinter, S., Robinson, J.S.:** Foetal respiratory movements, electrocortical and cardiovascular responses to hypoxaemia and hypercapnea in sheep. J. Physiol. 243:599, 1974.

2 **Boddy, K., Dawes, G.S., Fischer, R.L., Pinter, S., Robinson, J.S.:** The effects of pentobarbitone and pethidine on foetal breathing movements in sheep. Br. J. Pharmacol. 57:311, 1976.

3 **Fox, H.E., Steinbrecher, M., Pessel, D., Inglis, D., Medvid, L., Angel, E.:** Maternal ethanol ingestion and the occurrence of human fetal breathing movements. Am. J. Obstet. Gynecol. 132:354, 1978.

4 **Manning, F.A., Platt, L.D.:** Fetal breathing movements and the abnormal contraction stress test. Am. J. Obstet. Gynecol. 133:590, 1979.

5 **Manning, F.A., Platt, L.D., Sipos, L.:** Antepartum fetal evaluation: Development of a fetal biophysical profile. Am. J. Obstet. Gynecol. 136:787, 1980.

6 **Manning, F.A., Platt, L.D., Sipos, L., Keegan, K.A.:** Fetal breathing movements and the nonstress test in high-risk pregnancies. Am. J. Obstet. Gynecol. 135:511, 1979.

7 **Manning, F.A., Wyn Pugh, E., Boddy, K.:** Effect of cigarette smoking on fetal breathing movements in normal pregnancies. Br. Med. J. 1:551, 1975.

8 **Patrick, J., Campbell, K., Carmichael, L., Natale, K., Richardson, B.:** Patterns of human fetal breathing during the last 10 weeks of pregnancy. Obstet. Gynecol. 56:24, 1980.

9 **Patrick, J.E., Dalton, K.J., Dawes, G.S.:** Breathing patterns before death in fetal lambs. Am. J. Obstet. Gynecol. 125:73, 1976.

10 **Roberts, A.B., Little, D., Cooper, D., Campbell, S.:** Normal patterns of fetal activity in the third trimester. Br. J. Obstet. Gynecol. 86:4, 1979.

11 **Roberts, A.B., Stubbs, S.M., Mooney, R., Cooper, D., Brudenell, J.M., Campbell, S.:** Fetal activity in pregnancies complicated by maternal diabetes mellitus. Br. J. Obstet. Gynaecol. 87:485, 1980.

12 **Sadovsky, E., Polishuk, W.Z.:** Fetal movements in utero: Nature, assessment, prognostic value, timing of delivery. Obstet. Gynecol. 50:49, 1977.

13 **Sadovsky, E., Yaffe, H.:** Daily fetal movement recording and fetal prognosis. Obstet. Gynecol. 41:845, 1973.

Ultrasound in Ovarian Evaluation

10

In the past 10 years some of the mystery of ovarian function has been unraveled with the emergence of radioimmunoassays for various hormones which the ovary produces and to which it can respond. It has only been in the last 3 years, however, that the anatomy of the functioning ovary has been successfully studied. Dynamic ovarian events such as follicle maturation and ovulation can be sequentially observed with ultrasound.

Techniques

Since the ovary is often hidden by bowel and omentum, it is extremely important to carry out the ultrasound scan with a full bladder. This not only avails the operator of an ultrasound window, but it prevents the superimposition of abdominal contents between the transducer and the flattened-out adnexal structures.

A static scanner is sufficient for ovarian scanning. However, in order to fully outline the pelvic structures, the transducer must be swept in wide overlapping arcs. In this way both ovaries, pedicles, and the pelvic side walls (with the iliopsoas muscles) can be visualized. Sector scanners are ideal for ovarian scanning, since the laterally placed ovary can be examined from the midline using the bladder as a window. The linear array does not show the ovaries easily. A combination of parasagittal and transverse slices is required to fully evaluate follicular or ovarian volume. Hackelöer et al. (3) suggest that a series of sagittal scans be accomplished using the ovarian artery and vein as reference points. We have often been content to perform transverse sector scans through the pelvis so that both ovaries can be seen simultaneously (Figures 1 and 2). The largest diameters noted in the transverse plane should often suffice for quantitative assessment of ovarian or follicular size, but volumetric analysis requires a superior-inferior diameter that can only be obtained with parasagittal scans.

Normal ovulation

Various steroid hormones have been used to identify events within the menstrual cycle. For example, as the follicle develops estradiol (E_2) levels increase. Just

Figure 1

Transverse scan showing right ovary with two developing follicles.

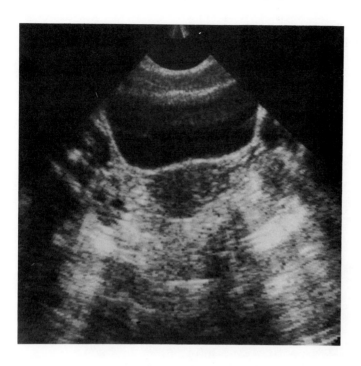

before ovulation there is a sudden spike in luteinizing hormone (LH) production. The adequacy of the luteal phase may be assessed by measurements of serum progesterone.

Thus far, reports correlating dominant follicular dimensions with estradiol levels demonstrate a parallel relationship during the preovulatory portion of the cycle. A range of mean follicular diameters at ovulation has been reported between 1.28 cm and 2.5 cm. Although most reports show a mean diameter of 2 to 2.5 cm, no single figure has been found to be an invariable predictor of ovulation, so that ultrasound alone cannot be used to accurately predict this event. Ultrasound in combination with estradiol levels, however, is particularly useful in following development of the follicle. Two studies (7, 8) show a consistent follicular growth of about 3 mm per day until the last preovulatory 24 hrs., during which time there is a sudden increase in diameter. A recent study validates ultrasound measurements of follicle size by correlation with aspirated follicular fluid volumes at the time of postultrasound laparoscopy.

Characterizing ovarian events during the luteal phase has been more difficult, and the inconsistent results

Figure 2

Transverse scan showing left ovary with small physiological cyst.

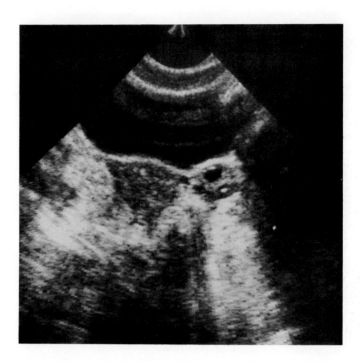

simply demonstrate the wide variety of changes that can occur. Queenan et al. (7) have described four different types of ultrasound appearances of the corpus luteum, ranging from *a small irregular regressive tendency* to a large (2 to 4 cm) corpus luteum cyst that may persist into the next cycle (Figure 3). DeCrespigny et al. (2) "observed" follicular rupture by rapid and frequent contact scanning of four patients at hourly intervals. This event occurred 28 to 35 hrs. after an LH peak in their patients. In two women there was rapid decrease in follicular volume followed by a gradual collapse of the follicle over a 35-min. period. Corpora hemorrhagica developed within 1 hr. of ovulation.

Ovulation induction

Most studies have demonstrated that Clomid-stimulated follicles are larger than the follicles of spontaneous ovulation by 2 to 3 mm. Estradiol levels are correspondingly higher. In one study (10) involving 20 induced cycles, pregnancy only occurred when follicular diameter exceeded 1.5 mm and serum E_2 levels were greater than 950 pmoles/liter.

Human menopausal gonadotropin (HMG) has been used as an exogenous source of follicle-stimulating hormone (FSH) along with human chorionic gonadotropin (hCG) to stimulate ovulation. Ultrasound

Figure 3

Transverse scan of the pelvis showing hemorrhagic corpus luteum.

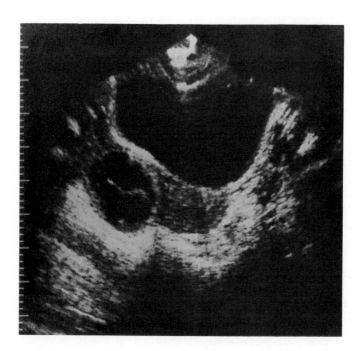

is particularly useful in managing HMG patients. If several large follicles are seen during HMG administration, hCG can be withheld to avoid the possibility of multiple gestation. Also, although few data are yet available regarding the early ultrasound findings of ovarian hyperstimulation, by following ovarian follicular number and size along with serum levels of estradiol, it is reasonable to assume that one could avoid this potentially hazardous syndrome by withholding hCG administration.

Infertile patients with high prolactin levels often ovulate only when exposed to bromocryptine. At Yale-New Haven Hospital, 18 bromocryptine-treated ovulatory cycles were studied by ultrasound (4). It was of interest that bilateral ovarian enlargement always occurred secondary to the development of follicles in both ovaries. The follicles were significantly larger than non-stimulated follicles (mean 2.7 cm in treated group compared with 1.8 mm in controls). Often the ovaries appeared similar to those stimulated by HMG.

Monitoring ovarian morphometry in cycles resulting in pregnancy

From data correlating basal body temperatures and hormonal indicators of ovulation (estradiol and LH peaks) with progesterone levels in late cycle, it is clear that not all cycles ending in menstruation are truly "normal." In work at Yale (6), about 36% of normal women with apparently normal cycles had follicles of small size and diminished E_2 levels. Furthermore, a Chilean investigator (9) has demonstrated differences in follicular growth in patients who become pregnant compared with those who do not.

It seems plausible that ultrasound monitoring is particularly useful in the management of infertile couples with regard to the timing of intercourse, the utility of medication, and the avoidance of therapeutic complications.

In vitro fertilization

From early work in this field there is no doubt that anything less than a total commitment on the part of a group venturing into the techniques of in vitro fertilization will be met with failure. There are many variables involved that require highly skilled personnel and the most up-to-date equipment. The Australian group (1) which has had the most success in this endeavor depends heavily upon ultrasound information derived originally from a comprehensive study of women with normal and stimulated ovulation. This team serially monitors follicular size and 24-hr. urine estrogen levels until a diameter of 1.7 cm and 30 ug/ ml, respectively, are attained, at which time the patients are hospitalized and LH levels are closely followed. Ultrasound evaluation just prior to laparoscopy allows the operator to select a dominant "ripe" follicle for aspiration. Furthermore, we have found that an ultrasound examination performed minutes before laparoscopy may save the patient from an unnecessary procedure if follicle rupture is shown to have already occurred.

Preliminary investigation in Copenhagen by Lenz et al. (5) suggests that it may be possible to aspirate eggs from preovulatory follicles under ultrasound direction. This would obviate the need for anesthesia and laparoscopy in in vitro fertilization. This group uses a linear array transducer with a special attachment to allow simultaneous viewing of the aspirating needle.

It is impossible to predict fully the future of in vitro fertilization, but there is no doubt that ultrasound must play a major role in its development.

References

1   **DeCrespigny, L.J. Ch., O'Herlihy, C., Hoult, I.J., Robinson, H.P.:** Ultrasound in an in vitro fertilization program. Fertil. Steril. 35:25, 1981.

2 **DeCrespigny, L. Ch., O'Herlihy, C., Robinson, H.P.:** Ultrasonic observation of the mechanism of human ovulation. Am. J. Obstet. Gynecol. 139:636, 1981.

3 **Hackelöer, B.J., Fleming, R., Robinson, H.P., Adam, A.H., Coutts, J.R.T.:** Correlation of ultrasonic and endocrinologic assessment of human follicular development. Am. J. Obstet. Gynecol. 135:122, 1979.

4 **Kort, H., Hobbins, J., DeCherney, A., Kase, N., Caldwell, B.V.:** Ovarian function and morphology following treatment with bromergocriptine. Unpublished data.

5 **Lenz, S., Lauritser, J.G., Kjellow, M.:** Collection of human oocytes for in vitro fertilization by ultrasonically-guided follicular puncture. 4th Annual Renier-Degraff Symposium, Nijmegen, Holland, August 20–22, 1981.

6 **Polan, M.L., Tortora, M., Caldwell, B.V., DeCherney, A.H., Haseltine, F.P., Kase, N.:** Abnormal ovarian cycles as diagnosed by ultrasound and serum estradiol levels. Fertil. Steril. 37:342, 1982.

7 **Queenan, J.T., O'Brien, G.D., Bains, L.M., Simpson, J., Collins, W.P., Campbell, S.:** Ultrasound scanning of ovaries to detect ovulation in women. Fertil. Steril. 34:99, 1980.

8 **Renaud, R.L., Macler, J., Dervain, I., Ehret, M.C., Aron, C., Plas-Roser, S., Spira, A., Pollack, H.:** Echographic study of follicular maturation and ovulation during the normal menstrual cycle. Fertil. Steril. 33:272, 1980.

9 **Serra, F.:** Santiago, Chile; Personal communication.

10 **Smith, D.H., Picker, R.H., Sinosich, M., Saunders, D.M.:** Assessment of ovulation by ultrasound and estradiol levels during spontaneous and induced cycles. Fertil. Steril. 33:387, 1980.

Appendix

This appendix has been included to assist the reader in rapidly determining fetal age and weight from a variety of published formulas. We have also included several graphs and nomograms which we hope will be useful in the antenatal management of women with problem pregnancies.

Figure 1

Crown-rump measurement as a determinant of fetal age. This determination is a useful and sensitive indicator of gestational age. In very
early pregnancy some patience is required to obtain the proper plane
for measurement.

From Robinson, H.P., Fleming J.E.E.: A critical evaluation of sonar
"crown-rump length" measurements. Br. J. Obstet. Gynaecol. 82:702,
1975.

Menstrual Maturity (weeks + days)	CRL (mm) Mean	CRL (mm) 2 S.D.	Menstrual Maturity (weeks + days)	CRL (mm) Mean	CRL (mm) 2 S.D.
6 + 2	7.0	3.3	10 + 0	33.0	7.2
6 + 3	6.5	1.4	10 + 1	33.8	7.6
6 + 4	7.0	4.6	10 + 2	35.2	7.3
6 + 5	6.5	4.2	10 + 3	36.0	7.9
6 + 6	10.0	2.6	10 + 4	37.3	9.7
7 + 0	9.3	2.3	10 + 5	43.4	7.7
7 + 1	10.3	8.0	10 + 6	40.1	7.1
7 + 2	11.8	5.7	11 + 0	46.7	6.1
7 + 3	12.8	4.8	11 + 1	43.6	7.2
7 + 4	13.4	6.7	11 + 2	47.5	6.2
7 + 5	15.4	3.6	11 + 3	48.8	5.9
7 + 6	15.4	4.4	11 + 4	49.0	9.5
8 + 0	17.0	4.9	11 + 5	54.0	9.8
8 + 1	19.5	5.7	11 + 6	56.2	9.5
8 + 2	19.4	6.2	12 + 0	58.3	9.4
8 + 3	20.4	5.0	12 + 1	56.8	7.2
8 + 4	21.3	3.8	12 + 2	59.4	6.6
8 + 5	20.9	2.4	12 + 3	62.6	8.6
8 + 6	23.2	3.6	12 + 4	63.5	9.5
9 + 0	25.8	6.0	12 + 5	67.7	6.4
9 + 1	25.4	4.6	12 + 6	66.5	8.2
9 + 2	26.7	4.4	13 + 0	72.5	4.2
9 + 3	27.0	2.8	13 + 1	69.7	8.5
9 + 4	32.5	4.2	13 + 2	73.0	15.1
9 + 5	30.0	10.0	13 + 3	77.0	8.5
9 + 6	31.3	5.5	13 + 4	—	—
			13 + 5	—	—
			13 + 6	76.0	5.7
			14 + 0	79.6	7.8

Figure 2

Days required to reach the discriminatory β-HCG zone (lower limit of normal).

From Kadar, N., Romero, R.: The timing of a repeat ultrasound examination in the evaluation for ectopic pregnancy. J. Clin. Ultrasound. 10:5, 1982.

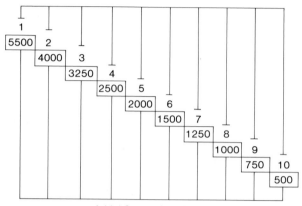

Initial Serum β-hCG Value

Figure 3

Yale nomogram for BPD using leading edge to leading edge; based on
B-mode dots (graticule).

Cm	Weeks Gestation	Cm	Weeks Gestation	Cm	Weeks Gestation
		4.2	18.9	6.9	28.1
		4.3	19.4	7.0	28.6
		4.4	19.4	7.1	29.1
		4.5	19.9	7.3	29.6
		4.6	20.4	7.4	30.0
		4.7	20.4	7.5	30.6
1.9	11.6	4.8	20.9	7.6	31.0
2.0	11.6	4.9	21.3	7.7	31.5
2.1	12.1	5.0	21.3	7.8	32.0
2.2	12.6	5.1	21.8	7.9	32.5
2.3	12.6	5.2	22.3	8.0	33.0
2.4	13.1	5.3	22.3	8.2	33.5
2.5	13.6	5.4	22.8	8.3	34.0
2.6	13.6	5.5	23.3	8.4	34.4
2.7	14.1	5.6	23.3	8.5	35.0
2.8	14.6	5.7	23.8	8.6	35.4
2.9	14.6	5.8	24.3	8.8	35.9
3.0	15.0	5.9	24.3	8.9	36.4
3.1	15.5	6.0	24.7	9.0*	36.9
3.2	15.5	6.1	25.2	9.1*	37.3
3.3	16.0	6.2	25.2	9.2*	37.8
3.4	16.5	6.3	25.7	9.3*	38.3
3.5	16.5	6.4	26.2	9.4*	38.8
3.6	17.0	6.5	26.2	9.6*	39.3
3.7	17.5	6.6	26.7	9.7*	39.8
3.8	17.9	6.7	27.2		
4.0	18.4	6.8	27.6		

* Indicates a fetus of 36 weeks or greater in a non-diabetic.

Figure 4

Nomogram for BPD using leading to falling edge

From Brown, R.E.: *Ultrasonography: Basic Principles and Clinical Application.* Warren H. Green, Inc., St. Louis.

mm	Weeks Gestation	mm	Weeks Gestation	mm	Weeks Gestation
23	13.1	49	19.5	75	29.0
24	13.3	50	19.8	76	29.4
25	13.5	51	20.1	77	29.9
26	13.7	52	20.4	78	30.4
27	13.9	53	20.7	79	30.8
28	14.1	54	21.0	80	31.3
29	14.3	55	21.4	81	31.8
30	14.6	56	21.7	82	32.3
31	14.8	57	22.0	83	32.8
32	15.0	58	22.4	84	33.3
33	15.3	59	22.7	85	33.8
34	15.5	60	23.1	86	34.3
35	15.7	61	23.4	87	34.8
36	16.0	62	23.8	88	35.4
37	16.2	63	24.1	89	35.9
38	16.5	64	24.5	90	36.5 mature
39	16.7	65	24.9	91	37.0
40	17.0	66	25.3	92	37.6
41	17.2	67	25.7	93	38.2
42	17.5	68	26.1	94	38.8
43	17.8	69	26.5	95	39.4
44	18.0	70	26.9	96	40.0
45	18.3	71	27.3	97	40.6
46	18.6	72	27.7	98	41.2
47	18.9	73	28.1	99	41.9
48	19.2	74	28.6	100	42.5

Figure 5

Nomogram for BPD: composite

From Kurtz, A.B., Wapner, R.J., Kurtz, R.J., Dershaw, D.D., Rubin, C.S., Cole-Beuglet, C., Goldberg, B.B.: Analysis of biparietal diameter as an accurate indicator of gestational age. J. Clin. Ultrasound 8:319–326, 1980.

mm	Weeks with Variation	mm	Weeks with Variation
20	12.0	60	22.3 to 25.5
21	12.0	61	22.6 to 25.8
22	12.2 to 13.2	62	23.1 to 26.1
23	12.4 to 13.6	63	23.4 to 26.4
24	12.6 to 13.8	64	23.8 to 26.8
25	12.9 to 14.1	65	24.1 to 27.1
26	13.1 to 14.3	66	24.5 to 27.5
27	13.4 to 14.6	67	25.0 to 27.8
28	13.6 to 15.0	68	25.3 to 28.1
29	13.9 to 15.2	69	25.8 to 28.4
30	14.1 to 15.5	70	26.3 to 28.7
31	14.3 to 15.9	71	26.7 to 29.1
32	14.5 to 16.1	72	27.2 to 29.4
33	14.7 to 16.5	73	27.6 to 29.8
34	15.0 to 16.8	74	28.1 to 30.1
35	15.2 to 17.2	75	28.5 to 30.5
36	15.4 to 17.4	76	29.0 to 31.0
37	15.6 to 17.8	77	29.2 to 31.4
38	15.9 to 18.1	78	29.6 to 32.0
39	16.1 to 18.5	79	29.9 to 32.5
40	16.4 to 18.8	80	30.2 to 33.0
41	16.5 to 19.3	81	30.7 to 33.5
42	16.6 to 19.8	82	31.2 to 34.0
43	16.8 to 20.2	83	31.5 to 34.5
44	16.9 to 20.7	84	31.9 to 35.1
45	17.0 to 21.2	85	32.3 to 35.7
46	17.4 to 21.4	86	32.8 to 36.2
47	17.8 to 21.6	87	33.4 to 36.6
48	18.2 to 21.8	88	33.9 to 37.1
49	18.6 to 22.0	89	34.6 to 37.6
50	19.0 to 22.2	90	35.1 to 38.1
51	19.3 to 22.5	91	35.9 to 38.5
52	19.5 to 22.9	92	36.7 to 38.9
53	19.8 to 23.2	93	37.3 to 39.3
54	20.1 to 23.7	94	37.9 to 40.1
55	20.4 to 24.0	95	38.5 to 40.9
56	20.7 to 24.3	96	39.1 to 41.5
57	21.1 to 24.5	97	39.9 to 42.1
58	21.5 to 24.9	98	40.5 to 43.1
59	21.9 to 25.1		

* Recommended biparietal diameter to gestational age based on the calculated weighted least-mean-squares-fit equation and 90% variation of the 17 studies.

Figure 6

Predicted BPD and weeks gestation from the inner and outer orbital diameters.

Adapted from Mayden, K.L., Tortora, M., Berkowitz, R.L., Bracken, M., Hobbins, J.C.: Orbital diameters: A new parameter for prenatal diagnosis and dating. Am. J. Obstet. Gynecol. 144:289–297, 1982.

BPD (cm)	Weeks Gestation	IOD (cm)	OOD (cm)	BPD (cm)	Weeks Gestation	IOD (cm)	OOD (cm)
1.9	11.6	0.5	1.3	5.8	24.3	1.6	4.1
2.0	11.6	0.5	1.4	5.9	24.3	1.6	4.2
2.1	12.1	0.6	1.5	6.0	24.7	1.6	4.3
2.2	12.6	0.6	1.6	6.1	25.2	1.6	4.3
2.3	12.6	0.6	1.7	6.2	25.2	1.6	4.4
2.4	13.1	0.7	1.7	6.3	25.7	1.7	4.4
2.5	13.6	0.7	1.8	6.4	26.2	1.7	4.5
2.6	13.6	0.7	1.9	6.5	26.2	1.7	4.5
2.7	14.1	0.8	2.0	6.6	26.7	1.7	4.6
2.8	14.6	0.8	2.1	6.7	27.2	1.7	4.6
2.9	14.6	0.8	2.1	6.8	27.6	1.7	4.7
3.0	15.0	0.9	2.2	6.9	28.1	1.7	4.7
3.1	15.5	0.9	2.3	7.0	28.6	1.8	4.8
3.2	15.5	0.9	2.4	7.1	29.1	1.8	4.8
3.3	16.0	1.0	2.5	7.3	29.6	1.8	4.9
3.4	16.5	1.0	2.5	7.4	30.0	1.8	5.0
3.5	16.5	1.0	2.6	7.5	30.6	1.8	5.0
3.6	17.0	1.0	2.7	7.6	31.0	1.8	5.1
3.7	17.5	1.1	2.7	7.7	31.5	1.8	5.1
3.8	17.9	1.1	2.8	7.8	32.0	1.8	5.2
4.0	18.4	1.2	3.0	7.9	32.5	1.9	5.2
4.2	18.9	1.2	3.1	8.0	33.0	1.9	5.3
4.3	19.4	1.2	3.2	8.2	33.5	1.9	5.4
4.4	19.4	1.3	3.2	8.3	34.0	1.9	5.4
4.5	19.9	1.3	3.3	8.4	34.4	1.9	5.4
4.6	20.4	1.3	3.4	8.5	35.0	1.9	5.5
4.7	20.4	1.3	3.4	8.6	35.4	1.9	5.5
4.8	20.9	1.4	3.5	8.8	35.9	1.9	5.6
4.9	21.3	1.4	3.6	8.9	36.4	1.9	5.6
5.0	21.3	1.4	3.6	9.0	36.9	1.9	5.7
5.1	21.8	1.4	3.7	9.1	37.3	1.9	5.7
5.2	22.3	1.4	3.8	9.2	37.8	1.9	5.8
5.3	22.3	1.5	3.8	9.3	38.3	1.9	5.8
5.4	22.8	1.5	3.9	9.4	38.8	1.9	5.8
5.5	23.3	1.5	4.0	9.6	39.3	1.9	5.9
5.6	23.3	1.5	4.0	9.7	39.8	1.9	5.9
5.7	23.8	1.5	4.1				

Calculated values from regression equation of bifrontal horn width: MEAN; Ventricular ratio; MEAN/BPD: Upper 95% confidence level (CL); and Upper 99% confidence level (CL)

From Denkhaus, H., Winsberg, F.: Ultrasonic measurement of the fetal ventricular system. Radiology 131:781–787, 1979.

BPD (cm)	MEAN (cm)	Ventricular Ratio	Upper 95% CL (cm)	Upper 99% CL (cm)
2.3	1.1	0.48	1.36	1.45
2.4	1.1	0.47	1.39	1.48
2.5	1.2	0.47	1.42	1.51
2.6	1.2	0.46	1.46	1.54
2.7	1.2	0.46	1.48	1.56
2.8	1.3	0.45	1.51	1.59
2.9	1.3	0.45	1.54	1.62
3.0	1.3	0.44	1.57	1.65
3.1	1.3	0.43	1.59	1.67
3.2	1.4	0.43	1.61	1.69
3.3	1.4	0.42	1.63	1.71
3.4	1.4	0.41	1.65	1.73
3.5	1.4	0.41	1.67	1.75
3.6	1.4	0.40	1.69	1.77
3.7	1.5	0.39	1.70	1.78
3.8	1.5	0.39	1.72	1.80
3.9	1.5	0.38	1.73	1.81
4.0	1.5	0.37	1.74	1.82
4.1	1.5	0.37	1.76	1.84
4.2	1.5	0.36	1.77	1.85
4.3	1.5	0.36	1.78	1.86
4.4	1.5	0.35	1.79	1.87
4.5	1.6	0.35	1.80	1.88
4.6	1.6	0.34	1.81	1.89
4.7	1.6	0.34	1.82	1.90
4.8	1.6	0.33	1.83	1.91
4.9	1.6	0.33	1.84	1.92
5.0	1.6	0.32	1.85	1.93
5.1	1.6	0.32	1.87	1.95
5.2	1.6	0.31	1.88	1.96
5.3	1.6	0.31	1.89	1.97
5.4	1.7	0.31	1.90	1.98
5.5	1.7	0.30	1.91	1.99
5.6	1.7	0.30	1.92	2.00
5.7	1.7	0.30	1.94	2.02
5.8	1.7	0.29	1.95	2.03
5.9	1.7	0.29	1.96	2.04
6.0	1.7	0.29	1.98	2.06
6.1	1.7	0.29	1.99	2.07
6.2	1.8	0.28	2.01	2.09
6.3	1.8	0.28	2.03	2.10
6.4	1.8	0.28	2.04	2.12
6.5	1.8	0.28	2.06	2.14
6.6	1.8	0.28	2.08	2.15
6.7	1.8	0.28	2.09	2.17
6.8	1.9	0.27	2.11	2.19
6.9	1.9	0.27	2.13	2.21
7.0	1.9	0.27	2.15	2.23
7.1	1.9	0.27	2.17	2.25
7.2	1.9	0.27	2.19	2.27
7.3	2.0	0.27	2.21	2.29
7.4	2.0	0.27	2.24	2.31
7.5	2.0	0.27	2.26	2.35
7.6	2.0	0.27	2.28	2.36
7.7	2.1	0.27	2.30	2.38
7.8	2.1	0.27	2.33	2.40
7.9	2.1	0.27	2.34	2.43
8.0	2.1	0.27	2.37	2.45
8.1	2.1	0.27	2.39	2.47
8.2	2.2	0.26	2.42	2.50
8.3	2.2	0.26	2.44	2.52
8.4	2.2	0.26	2.46	2.54
8.5	2.2	0.26	2.49	2.57
8.6	2.3	0.26	2.51	2.59
8.7	2.3	0.26	2.53	2.61
8.8	2.3	0.26	2.55	2.63
8.9	2.3	0.26	2.57	2.65
9.0	2.3	0.26	2.59	2.67
9.1	2.4	0.26	2.61	2.69
9.2	2.4	0.26	2.63	2.71
9.3	2.4	0.26	2.65	2.73
9.4	2.4	0.26	2.67	2.75
9.5	2.4	0.26	2.69	2.77
9.6	2.4	0.25	2.70	2.78
9.7	2.5	0.25	2.72	2.80
9.8	2.5	0.25	2.74	2.82
9.9	2.5	0.25	2.77	2.85
10.0	2.5	0.25	2.79	2.87

Figure 8

Abdominal circumference as a predictor of fetal weight. The circumference measurement is made at right angles to the fetal spine at the
level of the umbilical vein (Chapter 6) with a map reader.

From Campbell, S., Wilkin, D.: Ultrasonic measurement of fetal abdomen circumference in the estimation of fetal weight. Br. J. Obstet.
Gynaecol. 82:689, 1975.

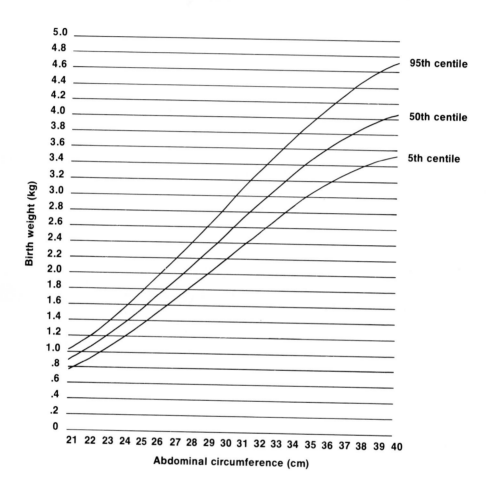

Figure 9

Abdominal circumference growth curve.

From Hobbins, J.C., Grannum, P.A.T., Berkowitz, R.L., Silverman, R., Mahoney, M.J.: Ultrasound in the diagnosis of congenital anomalies. Am. J. Obstet. Gynecol. 134:331, 1979.

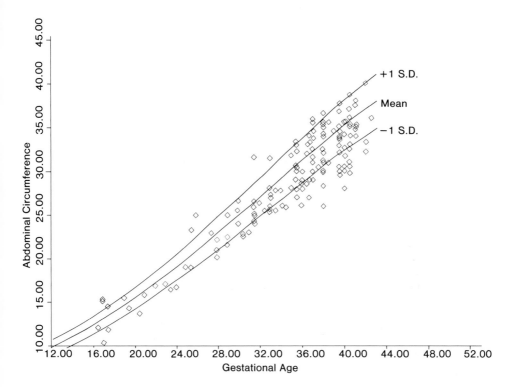

Figure 10

Mean fetal H:A circumference ratios with 5th and 95th centile limits related to menstrual age from 13 to 42 weeks; values have been combined into 2-weekly groupings to smooth out fluctuations due to small numbers (568 individual measurements).

From Campbell, S., Thoms, A. Ultrasound measurement of the fetal head-to-abdomen circumference ratio in assessment of growth retardation. Br. J. Obstet. Gynaecol. 84:165, 1977.

Menstrual Age (weeks)	Number of Measurements	H:A Circumference Ratio		
		5th Centile	Mean	95th Centile
13–14	18	1.14	1.23	1.31
15–16	39	1.05	1.22	1.39
17–18	77	1.07	1.18	1.29
19–20	54	1.09	1.18	1.26
21–22	41	1.06	1.15	1.25
23–24	22	1.05	1.13	1.21
25–26	18	1.04	1.13	1.22
27–28	36	1.05	1.13	1.22
29–30	23	0.99	1.10	1.21
31–32	31	0.96	1.07	1.17
33–34	42	0.96	1.04	1.11
35–36	49	0.93	1.02	1.11
37–38	67	0.92	0.98	1.05
39–40	47	0.87	0.97	1.06
41–42	4	0.93	0.96	1.00

Figure 11

Uterine volume: formula = length × width × thickness × 0.5233 (see Chapter 6).

From Gohari, P., Berkowitz, R.L., Hobbins, J.C.: Prediction of intrauterine growth retardation by determination of total intrauterine volume. Am. J. Obstet. Gynecol. 127:255, 1977.

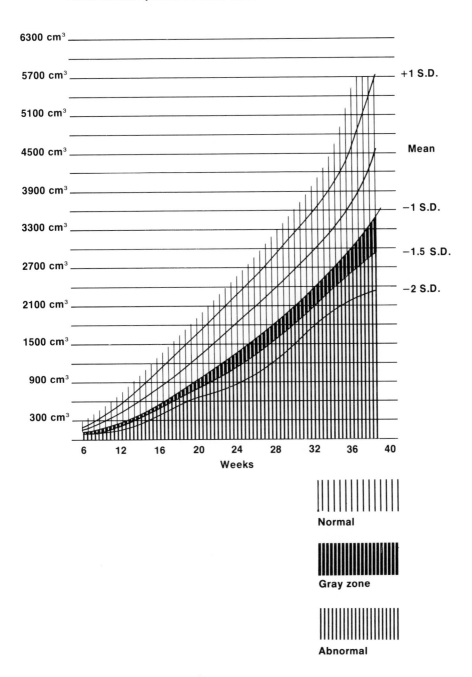

Figure 12

Estimated fetal weights: Log (birth weight) = −1.7492 + 0.166 (BPD) + 0.046 (AC) − 2.646 (AC × BPD)/1000.

From Shepard, J.J., Richards, V.A., Berkowitz, R.L., Warsof, S.L., Hobbins, J.C: An evaluation of two equations for predicting fetal weight by ultrasound. Am. J. Obstet. Gynecol. 142:47, 1982.

Biparietal diameters	Abdominal circumferences											
	15.5	16.0	16.5	17.0	17.5	18.0	18.5	19.0	19.5	20.0	20.5	21.0
3.1	224	234	244	255	267	279	291	304	318	332	346	362
3.2	231	241	251	263	274	286	299	312	326	340	355	371
3.3	237	248	259	270	282	294	307	321	335	349	365	381
3.4	244	255	266	278	290	302	316	329	344	359	374	391
3.5	251	262	274	285	298	311	324	338	353	368	384	401
3.6	259	270	281	294	306	319	333	347	362	378	394	411
3.7	266	278	290	302	315	328	342	357	372	388	404	422
3.8	274	286	298	310	324	337	352	366	382	398	415	432
3.9	282	294	306	319	333	347	361	376	392	409	426	444
4.0	290	303	315	328	342	356	371	386	403	419	437	455
4.1	299	311	324	338	352	366	381	397	413	430	448	467
4.2	308	320	333	347	361	376	392	408	424	442	460	479
4.3	317	330	343	357	371	387	402	419	436	453	472	491
4.4	326	339	353	367	382	397	413	430	447	465	484	504
4.5	335	349	363	377	393	408	425	442	459	478	497	517
4.6	345	359	373	388	404	420	436	454	472	490	510	530
4.7	355	369	384	399	415	431	448	466	484	503	523	544
4.8	366	380	395	410	426	443	460	478	497	517	537	558
4.9	376	391	406	422	438	455	473	491	510	530	551	572
5.0	387	402	418	434	451	468	486	505	524	544	565	587
5.1	399	414	430	446	463	481	499	518	538	559	580	602
5.2	410	426	442	459	476	494	513	532	552	573	595	618
5.3	422	438	455	472	489	508	527	547	567	589	611	634
5.4	435	451	468	485	503	522	541	561	582	604	627	650
5.5	447	464	481	499	517	536	556	577	598	620	643	667
5.6	461	477	495	513	532	551	571	592	614	636	660	684
5.7	474	491	509	527	547	566	587	608	630	653	677	701
5.8	488	505	524	542	562	582	603	625	647	670	695	719
5.9	502	520	539	558	578	598	619	642	664	688	713	738
6.0	517	535	554	573	594	615	636	659	682	706	731	757
6.1	532	550	570	590	610	632	654	677	700	725	750	777
6.2	547	566	586	606	627	649	672	695	719	744	770	797
6.3	563	583	603	624	645	667	690	714	738	764	790	817
6.4	580	600	620	641	663	686	709	733	758	784	811	838
6.5	597	617	638	659	682	705	728	753	778	805	832	860
6.6	614	635	656	678	701	724	748	773	799	826	853	882
6.7	632	653	675	697	720	744	769	794	820	848	876	905
6.8	651	672	694	717	740	765	790	816	842	870	898	928
6.9	670	691	714	737	761	786	811	838	865	893	922	952
7.0	689	711	734	758	782	807	833	860	888	916	946	976
7.1	709	732	755	779	804	830	856	883	912	941	971	1,002
7.2	730	763	777	801	827	853	880	907	936	965	996	1,027
7.3	751	775	799	824	850	876	904	932	961	991	1,022	1,054
7.4	773	797	822	847	874	901	928	957	987	1,017	1,049	1,081
7.5	796	820	845	871	898	925	954	983	1,013	1,044	1,076	1,109
7.6	819	844	870	896	923	951	980	1,009	1,040	1,072	1,104	1,137
7.7	843	868	894	921	949	977	1,007	1,037	1,068	1,100	1,133	1,167
7.8	868	894	920	947	975	1,004	1,034	1,065	1,096	1,129	1,162	1,197
7.9	893	919	946	974	1,003	1,032	1,062	1,094	1,126	1,159	1,193	1,228
8.0	919	946	973	1,002	1,031	1,061	1,091	1,123	1,156	1,189	1,224	1,259
8.1	946	973	1,001	1,030	1,060	1,090	1,121	1,153	1,187	1,221	1,256	1,292
8.2	974	1,001	1,030	1,059	1,089	1,120	1,152	1,185	1,218	1,253	1,288	1,325
8.3	1,002	1,030	1,059	1,089	1,120	1,151	1,183	1,217	1,251	1,286	1,322	1,359
8.4	1,032	1,060	1,090	1,120	1,151	1,183	1,216	1,249	1,284	1,320	1,356	1,394
8.5	1,062	1,091	1,121	1,151	1,183	1,216	1,249	1,283	1,318	1,355	1,392	1,430
8.6	1,093	1,122	1,153	1,184	1,216	1,249	1,283	1,318	1,354	1,390	1,428	1,467
8.7	1,125	1,155	1,186	1,218	1,250	1,284	1,318	1,353	1,390	1,427	1,465	1,505
8.8	1,157	1,188	1,220	1,252	1,285	1,319	1,354	1,390	1,427	1,465	1,504	1,543
8.9	1,191	1,222	1,254	1,287	1,321	1,356	1,391	1,428	1,465	1,503	1,543	1,583
9.0	1,226	1,258	1,290	1,324	1,358	1,393	1,429	1,456	1,504	1,543	1,583	1,624
9.1	1,262	1,294	1,327	1,361	1,396	1,432	1,468	1,506	1,544	1,584	1,624	1,666
9.2	1,299	1,332	1,365	1,400	1,435	1,471	1,508	1,546	1,586	1,626	1,667	1,709
9.3	1,337	1,370	1,404	1,439	1,475	1,512	1,550	1,588	1,628	1,668	1,710	1,753
9.4	1,376	1,410	1,444	1,480	1,516	1,554	1,592	1,631	1,671	1,712	1,755	1,798
9.5	1,416	1,450	1,486	1,522	1,559	1,597	1,635	1,675	1,716	1,758	1,800	1,844
9.6	1,457	1,492	1,528	1,565	1,602	1,641	1,680	1,720	1,762	1,804	1,847	1,892
9.7	1,500	1,535	1,572	1,609	1,547	1,686	1,726	1,767	1,809	1,852	1,895	1,940
9.8	1,544	1,580	1,617	1,654	1,693	1,733	1,773	1,815	1,857	1,900	1,945	1,990
9.9	1,589	1,625	1,663	1,701	1,740	1,781	1,822	1,864	1,907	1,951	1,996	2,042
10.0	1,635	1,672	1,710	1,749	1,789	1,830	1,871	1,914	1,958	2,002	2,048	2,094

SD = ±106.0 gm/kg of birth weight.

Figure 12—*Continued*

					Abdominal circumferences							
21.5	22.0	22.5	23.0	23.5	24.0	24.5	25.0	25.5	26.0	26.5	27.0	27.5
378	395	412	431	450	470	491	513	536	559	584	610	638
388	405	423	441	461	481	502	525	548	572	597	624	651
397	415	433	452	472	493	514	537	560	585	611	638	666
408	425	444	463	483	504	526	549	573	598	624	652	680
418	436	455	475	495	517	539	562	587	612	638	666	695
429	447	466	486	507	529	552	575	600	626	653	681	710
440	458	478	498	519	542	565	589	614	640	667	696	725
451	470	490	510	532	554	578	602	628	654	682	711	741
462	482	502	523	545	568	592	616	642	669	697	727	757
474	494	514	536	558	581	606	631	657	684	713	743	773
486	506	527	549	572	595	620	645	672	700	729	759	790
498	519	540	562	585	609	634	660	688	716	745	776	807
511	532	554	576	600	624	649	676	703	732	762	793	825
524	545	567	590	614	639	665	692	719	749	779	810	843
538	559	581	605	629	654	680	708	736	765	796	828	861
551	573	596	620	644	670	696	724	753	783	814	846	880
565	588	611	635	660	686	713	741	770	801	832	865	899
580	602	626	650	676	702	730	758	788	819	851	884	919
594	617	641	666	692	719	747	776	806	837	870	903	938
610	633	657	683	709	736	765	794	824	856	889	923	959
625	649	674	699	726	754	783	812	843	876	909	944	980
641	665	690	717	744	772	801	831	863	895	929	964	1,001
657	682	708	734	762	790	820	851	883	916	950	986	1,023
674	699	725	752	780	809	839	870	903	936	971	1,007	1,045
691	717	743	771	799	828	859	891	924	958	993	1,030	1,068
709	735	762	789	818	848	879	911	945	979	1,015	1,052	1,091
727	753	780	809	838	869	900	933	966	1,001	1,038	1,075	1,114
745	772	800	829	858	889	921	954	989	1,024	1,061	1,099	1,139
764	792	820	849	879	911	943	977	1,011	1,047	1,085	1,123	1,163
784	811	840	870	900	932	965	999	1,035	1,071	1,109	1,148	1,189
804	832	861	891	922	955	988	1,023	1,058	1,095	1,134	1,173	1,214
824	853	882	913	945	977	1,011	1,046	1,083	1,120	1,159	1,199	1,241
845	874	904	935	967	1,001	1,035	1,071	1,107	1,145	1,185	1,226	1,268
867	896	927	958	991	1,025	1,059	1,096	1,133	1,171	1,211	1,253	1,295
889	919	950	982	1,015	1,049	1,084	1,121	1,159	1,198	1,238	1,280	1,323
911	942	973	1,006	1,039	1,074	1,110	1,147	1,185	1,225	1,266	1,308	1,352
935	965	997	1,030	1,065	1,100	1,136	1,174	1,213	1,253	1,294	1,337	1,381
958	990	1,022	1,056	1,090	1,126	1,163	1,201	1,241	1,281	1,323	1,367	1,411
983	1,015	1,048	1,082	1,117	1,153	1,190	1,229	1,269	1,310	1,353	1,397	1,442
1,008	1,040	1,074	1,108	1,144	1,181	1,219	1,258	1,298	1,340	1,383	1,427	1,473
1,033	1,066	1,100	1,135	1,171	1,209	1,247	1,287	1,328	1,370	1,414	1,459	1,505
1,060	1,093	1,128	1,163	1,200	1,238	1,277	1,317	1,358	1,401	1,445	1,491	1,538
1,087	1,121	1,156	1,192	1,229	1,267	1,307	1,348	1,390	1,433	1,478	1,524	1,571
1,114	1,149	1,184	1,221	1,259	1,297	1,338	1,379	1,421	1,465	1,511	1,557	1,605
1,143	1,178	1,214	1,251	1,289	1,328	1,369	1,411	1,454	1,499	1,544	1,592	1,640
1,172	1,207	1,244	1,281	1,320	1,360	1,401	1,444	1,487	1,533	1,579	1,627	1,676
1,202	1,238	1,275	1,313	1,352	1,393	1,434	1,477	1,522	1,567	1,614	1,663	1,712
1,232	1,269	1,306	1,345	1,385	1,426	1,468	1,512	1,557	1,603	1,650	1,699	1,749
1,264	1,301	1,339	1,378	1,418	1,460	1,503	1,547	1,592	1,639	1,687	1,737	1,787
1,296	1,333	1,372	1,412	1,453	1,495	1,538	1,583	1,629	1,676	1,725	1,775	1,826
1,329	1,367	1,406	1,446	1,488	1,531	1,575	1,620	1,666	1,714	1,763	1,814	1,866
1,363	1,401	1,441	1,482	1,524	1,567	1,612	1,657	1,704	1,753	1,803	1,854	1,906
1,397	1,436	1,477	1,518	1,561	1,605	1,650	1,696	1,744	1,793	1,843	1,895	1,948
1,433	1,473	1,513	1,555	1,599	1,643	1,689	1,735	1,784	1,833	1,884	1,936	1,990
1,469	1,510	1,551	1,594	1,637	1,682	1,728	1,776	1,825	1,875	1,926	1,979	2,033
1,507	1,548	1,589	1,633	1,677	1,722	1,769	1,817	1,866	1,917	1,969	2,022	2,077
1,545	1,586	1,629	1,673	1,717	1,764	1,811	1,859	1,909	1,960	2,013	2,067	2,122
1,584	1,626	1,669	1,714	1,759	1,806	1,854	1,903	1,953	2,005	2,058	2,113	2,169
1,625	1,667	1,711	1,756	1,802	1,849	1,897	1,947	1,998	2,050	2,104	2,159	2,216
1,666	1,709	1,753	1,799	1,845	1,893	1,942	1,992	2,044	2,097	2,151	2,207	2,264
1,708	1,752	1,797	1,843	1,890	1,938	1,988	2,039	2,091	2,144	2,199	2,255	2,313
1,752	1,796	1,841	1,888	1,936	1,984	2,035	2,086	2,139	2,193	2,248	2,305	2,363
1,796	1,841	1,887	1,934	1,982	2,032	2,083	2,135	2,188	2,242	2,298	2,356	2,414
1,842	1,887	1,934	1,982	2,030	2,080	2,132	2,184	2,238	2,293	2,350	2,407	2,467
1,889	1,935	1,982	2,030	2,080	2,130	2,182	2,235	2,289	2,345	2,402	2,460	2,520
1,937	1,984	2,031	2,080	2,130	2,181	2,233	2,287	2,342	2,398	2,456	2,515	2,575
1,986	2,033	2,082	2,131	2,181	2,233	2,286	2,340	2,396	2,452	2,510	2,570	2,631
2,037	2,085	2,133	2,183	2,234	2,286	2,340	2,395	2,451	2,508	2,567	2,627	2,688
2,089	2,137	2,186	2,237	2,288	2,341	2,395	2,450	2,507	2,565	2,624	2,684	2,746
2,142	2,191	2,241	2,292	2,344	2,397	2,452	2,507	2,564	2,623	2,682	2,743	2,806

Figure 12—*Continued*

Biparietal diameters	Abdominal circumferences											
	28.0	28.5	29.0	29.5	30.0	30.5	31.0	31.5	32.0	32.5	33.0	33.5
3.1	666	696	726	759	793	828	865	903	943	985	1,029	1,075
3.2	680	710	742	774	809	844	882	921	961	1,004	1,048	1,094
3.3	695	725	757	790	825	861	899	938	979	1,022	1,067	1,114
3.4	710	740	773	806	841	878	916	956	998	1,041	1,087	1,134
3.5	725	756	789	823	858	896	934	975	1,017	1,061	1,107	1,154
3.6	740	772	805	840	876	913	953	993	1,036	1,080	1,127	1,175
3.7	756	788	822	857	893	931	971	1,012	1,056	1,101	1,147	1,196
3.8	772	805	839	874	911	950	990	1,032	1,076	1,121	1,168	1,218
3.9	789	822	856	892	930	969	1,009	1,052	1,096	1,142	1,190	1,240
4.0	806	839	874	911	949	988	1,029	1,072	1,117	1,163	1,212	1,262
4.1	828	857	892	929	968	1,008	1,049	1,093	1,138	1,185	1,234	1,285
4.2	841	875	911	948	987	1,028	1,070	1,114	1,159	1,207	1,256	1,308
4.3	859	893	930	968	1,007	1,048	1,091	1,135	1,181	1,229	1,279	1,331
4.4	877	912	949	987	1,027	1,069	1,112	1,157	1,204	1,252	1,303	1,355
4.5	896	932	969	1,008	1,048	1,090	1,134	1,179	1,226	1,275	1,326	1,380
4.6	915	951	989	1,028	1,069	1,112	1,156	1,202	1,249	1,299	1,351	1,404
4.7	934	971	1,010	1,049	1,091	1,134	1,178	1,225	1,273	1,323	1,375	1,430
4.8	954	992	1,031	1,071	1,113	1,156	1,201	1,248	1,297	1,348	1,401	1,455
4.9	975	1,013	1,052	1,093	1,135	1,179	1,225	1,272	1,322	1,373	1,426	1,482
5.0	996	1,034	1,074	1,115	1,158	1,203	1,249	1,297	1,347	1,399	1,452	1,508
5.1	1,017	1,056	1,096	1,138	1,181	1,226	1,273	1,322	1,372	1,425	1,479	1,535
5.2	1,039	1,078	1,119	1,161	1,205	1,251	1,298	1,347	1,398	1,451	1,506	1,563
5.3	1,061	1,101	1,142	1,185	1,229	1,276	1,323	1,373	1,425	1,478	1,533	1,591
5.4	1,084	1,124	1,166	1,209	1,254	1,301	1,349	1,399	1,452	1,506	1,562	1,620
5.5	1,107	1,148	1,190	1,234	1,279	1,327	1,376	1,426	1,479	1,534	1,590	1,649
5.6	1,131	1,172	1,215	1,259	1,305	1,353	1,402	1,454	1,507	1,562	1,619	1,678
5.7	1,155	1,197	1,240	1,285	1,332	1,380	1,430	1,482	1,535	1,591	1,649	1,709
5.8	1,180	1,222	1,266	1,311	1,358	1,407	1,458	1,510	1,564	1,621	1,679	1,739
5.9	1,205	1,248	1,292	1,338	1,386	1,435	1,486	1,539	1,594	1,651	1,710	1,770
6.0	1,231	1,274	1,319	1,366	1,414	1,464	1,515	1,569	1,624	1,682	1,741	1,802
6.1	1,257	1,301	1,346	1,393	1,442	1,493	1,545	1,599	1,655	1,713	1,773	1,835
6.2	1,284	1,328	1,374	1,422	1,471	1,522	1,575	1,630	1,686	1,745	1,805	1,868
6.3	1,311	1,356	1,403	1,451	1,501	1,552	1,606	1,661	1,718	1,777	1,838	1,901
6.4	1,339	1,385	1,432	1,481	1,531	1,583	1,637	1,693	1,751	1,810	1,872	1,935
6.5	1,368	1,414	1,462	1,511	1,562	1,615	1,669	1,725	1,784	1,844	1,906	1,970
6.6	1,397	1,444	1,492	1,542	1,594	1,647	1,702	1,759	1,817	1,878	1,941	2,006
6.7	1,427	1,474	1,523	1,574	1,626	1,679	1,735	1,792	1,852	1,913	1,976	2,042
6.8	1,458	1,505	1,555	1,606	1,658	1,713	1,769	1,827	1,887	1,949	2,012	2,078
6.9	1,489	1,537	1,587	1,639	1,692	1,747	1,803	1,862	1,922	1,985	2,049	2,116
7.0	1,521	1,570	1,620	1,672	1,726	1,781	1,839	1,898	1,959	2,022	2,087	2,154
7.1	1,553	1,603	1,654	1,706	1,761	1,817	1,875	1,934	1,996	2,059	2,125	2,193
7.2	1,586	1,636	1,688	1,741	1,796	1,853	1,911	1,971	2,044	2,098	2,164	2,232
7.3	1,620	1,671	1,723	1,777	1,832	1,890	1,948	2,009	2,072	2,137	2,203	2,272
7.4	1,655	1,706	1,759	1,813	1,869	1,927	1,987	2,048	2,111	2,176	2,244	2,313
7.5	1,690	1,742	1,795	1,850	1,907	1,965	2,025	2,087	2,151	2,217	2,265	2,354
7.6	1,727	1,779	1,833	1,888	1,945	2,004	2,065	2,127	2,192	2,258	2,326	2,397
7.7	1,764	1,816	1,871	1,927	1,985	2,044	2,105	2,168	2,233	2,300	2,369	2,440
7.8	1,801	1,855	1,910	1,966	2,025	2,085	2,146	2,210	2,275	2,343	2,412	2,484
7.9	1,840	1,894	1,949	2,006	2,065	2,126	2,188	2,252	2,318	2,386	2,456	2,528
8.0	1,879	1,934	1,990	2,048	2,107	2,168	2,231	2,296	2,362	2,431	2,501	2,574
8.1	1,919	1,975	2,031	2,089	2,149	2,211	2,275	2,340	2,407	2,476	2,547	2,620
8.2	1,960	2,016	2,073	2,132	2,193	2,255	2,319	2,385	2,462	2,522	2,594	2,667
8.3	2,002	2,059	2,116	2,176	2,237	2,300	2,364	2,431	2,499	2,569	2,641	2,715
8.4	2,045	2,102	2,160	2,220	2,282	2,345	2,410	2,477	2,546	2,617	2,689	2,764
8.5	2,089	2,146	2,205	2,266	2,328	2,392	2,457	2,525	2,594	2,665	2,739	2,814
8.6	2,134	2,192	2,251	2,312	2,375	2,439	2,505	2,573	2,643	2,715	2,789	2,864
8.7	2,179	2,238	2,298	2,359	2,423	2,488	2,554	2,623	2,693	2,765	2,840	2,916
8.8	2,226	2,285	2,346	2,408	2,472	2,537	2,604	2,673	2,744	2,817	2,892	2,968
8.9	2,274	2,333	2,394	2,457	2,521	2,587	2,655	2,725	2,796	2,869	2,944	3,021
9.0	2,322	2,382	2,444	2,507	2,572	2,639	2,707	2,777	2,849	2,923	2,998	3,076
9.1	2,372	2,433	2,495	2,559	2,624	2,691	2,760	2,830	2,903	2,977	3,053	3,131
9.2	2,423	2,484	2,547	2,611	2,677	2,744	2,814	2,885	2,958	3,032	3,109	3,187
9.3	2,475	2,536	2,599	2,664	2,731	2,799	2,869	2,940	3,014	3,089	3,166	3,245
9.4	2,527	2,590	2,653	2,719	2,786	2,854	2,925	2,997	3,070	3,146	3,224	3,303
9.5	2,582	2,644	2,709	2,774	2,842	2,911	2,982	3,054	3,129	3,205	3,283	3,362
9.6	2,637	2,700	2,765	2,831	2,899	2,969	3,040	3,113	3,188	3,264	3,343	3,423
9.7	2,693	2,757	2,822	2,889	2,958	3,028	3,099	3,173	3,248	3,325	3,404	3,484
9.8	2,751	2,815	2,881	2,948	3,017	3,088	3,160	3,234	3,309	3,387	3,466	3,547
9.9	2,810	2,874	2,941	3,009	3,078	3,149	3,222	3,296	3,372	3,450	3,529	3,611
10.0	2,870	2,935	3,002	3,070	3,140	3,211	3,285	3,359	3,436	3,514	3,594	3,676

Figure 12—*Continued*

Abdominal circumferences												
34.0	34.5	35.0	35.5	36.0	36.5	37.0	37.5	38.0	38.5	39.0	39.5	40.0
1,123	1,173	1,225	1,279	1,336	1,396	1,458	1,523	1,591	1,661	1,735	1,812	1,893
1,143	1,193	1,246	1,301	1,358	1,418	1,481	1,546	1,615	1,686	1,761	1,838	1,920
1,163	1,214	1,267	1,323	1,381	1,441	1,504	1,570	1,639	1,711	1,786	1,865	1,946
1,183	1,235	1,289	1,345	1,403	1,464	1,528	1,595	1,664	1,737	1,812	1,891	1,973
1,204	1,256	1,311	1,367	1,426	1,488	1,552	1,619	1,689	1,762	1,839	1,918	2,001
1,226	1,278	1,333	1,390	1,450	1,512	1,577	1,645	1,715	1,789	1,865	1,945	2,029
1,247	1,300	1,356	1,413	1,474	1,536	1,602	1,670	1,741	1,815	1,893	1,973	2,057
1,269	1,323	1,379	1,437	1,498	1,561	1,627	1,696	1,768	1,842	1,920	2,001	2,086
1,292	1,346	1,402	1,461	1,523	1,586	1,653	1,722	1,794	1,870	1,948	2,030	2,115
1,315	1,369	1,426	1,486	1,548	1,612	1,679	1,749	1,822	1,898	1,977	2,059	2,145
1,338	1,393	1,451	1,511	1,573	1,638	1,706	1,776	1,849	1,926	2,005	2,088	2,174
1,361	1,417	1,475	1,536	1,599	1,664	1,733	1,804	1,878	1,954	2,035	2,118	2,205
1,385	1,442	1,500	1,562	1,625	1,691	1,760	1,832	1,906	1,984	2,064	2,148	2,236
1,410	1,467	1,526	1,588	1,652	1,718	1,788	1,860	1,935	2,013	2,094	2,179	2,267
1,435	1,492	1,552	1,614	1,679	1,746	1,816	1,889	1,964	2,043	2,125	2,210	2,298
1,460	1,518	1,579	1,641	1,706	1,774	1,845	1,918	1,994	2,073	2,156	2,241	2,330
1,486	1,545	1,605	1,669	1,734	1,803	1,874	1,948	2,024	2,104	2,187	2,273	2,363
1,512	1,571	1,633	1,697	1,763	1,832	1,904	1,978	2,055	2,136	2,219	2,306	2,396
1,539	1,599	1,661	1,725	1,792	1,861	1,934	2,009	2,086	2,167	2,251	2,339	2,429
1,566	1,626	1,689	1,754	1,821	1,891	1,964	2,040	2,118	2,200	2,284	2,372	2,463
1,594	1,655	1,718	1,783	1,851	1,922	1,995	2,071	2,150	2,232	2,317	2,406	2,498
1,622	1,683	1,747	1,813	1,882	1,953	2,027	2,103	2,183	2,266	2,351	2,440	2,532
1,651	1,713	1,777	1,843	1,913	1,984	2,059	2,136	2,216	2,299	2,386	2,475	2,568
1,680	1,742	1,807	1,874	1,944	2,016	2,091	2,169	2,250	2,333	2,420	2,510	2,604
1,710	1,773	1,838	1,906	1,976	2,049	2,124	2,203	2,284	2,368	2,456	2,546	2,640
1,740	1,803	1,869	1,938	2,008	2,082	2,158	2,237	2,319	2,403	2,491	2,582	2,677
1,770	1,835	1,901	1,970	2,041	2,115	2,192	2,272	2,354	2,439	2,528	2,619	2,714
1,802	1,866	1,934	2,003	2,075	2,150	2,227	2,307	2,390	2,475	2,564	2,657	2,752
1,834	1,899	1,966	2,037	2,109	2,184	2,262	2,342	2,426	2,512	2,602	2,694	2,790
1,866	1,932	2,000	2,071	2,144	2,219	2,298	2,379	2,463	2,550	2,640	2,733	2,829
1,899	1,965	2,034	2,105	2,179	2,255	2,334	2,416	2,500	2,588	2,678	2,772	2,869
1,932	1,999	2,069	2,140	2,215	2,291	2,371	2,453	2,538	2,626	2,717	2,811	2,909
1,967	2,034	2,104	2,176	2,251	2,328	2,408	2,491	2,577	2,665	2,757	2,851	2,949
2,001	2,069	2,140	2,213	2,288	2,366	2,446	2,530	2,616	2,705	2,797	2,892	2,991
2,037	2,105	2,176	2,250	2,326	2,404	2,485	2,569	2,656	2,745	2,838	2,933	3,032
2,073	2,142	2,213	2,287	2,364	2,443	2,524	2,609	2,696	2,786	2,879	2,975	3,075
2,109	2,179	2,251	2,326	2,403	2,482	2,564	2,649	2,737	2,827	2,921	3,018	3,117
2,147	2,217	2,290	2,365	2,442	2,522	2,605	2,690	2,778	2,869	2,964	3,061	3,161
2,184	2,255	2,329	2,404	2,482	2,563	2,646	2,732	2,821	2,912	3,007	3,104	3,205
2,223	2,295	2,368	2,444	2,523	2,604	2,688	2,774	2,863	2,955	3,050	3,149	3,250
2,262	2,334	2,409	2,485	2,564	2,646	2,730	2,817	2,907	2,999	3,095	3,193	3,295
2,302	2,375	2,450	2,527	2,607	2,689	2,773	2,861	2,951	3,044	3,140	3,239	3,341
2,343	2,416	2,491	2,569	2,649	2,732	2,817	2,905	2,996	3,089	3,186	3,285	3,388
2,384	2,458	2,534	2,612	2,693	2,776	2,862	2,950	3,041	3,135	3,232	3,332	3,435
2,426	2,501	2,577	2,656	2,737	2,821	2,907	2,996	3,088	3,182	3,279	3,380	3,483
2,469	2,544	2,621	2,700	2,782	2,866	2,953	3,042	3,134	3,229	3,327	3,428	3,531
2,513	2,588	2,666	2,746	2,828	2,912	3,000	3,090	3,182	3,277	3,376	3,477	3,581
2,557	2,633	2,711	2,792	2,874	2,959	3,047	3,137	3,230	3,326	3,425	3,526	3,631
2,603	2,679	2,757	2,838	2,921	3,007	3,095	3,186	3,279	3,376	3,475	3,576	3,681
2,649	2,725	2,804	2,886	2,969	3,056	3,144	3,235	3,329	3,426	3,525	3,627	3,733
2,695	2,773	2,852	2,934	3,018	3,105	3,194	3,286	3,380	3,477	3,577	3,679	3,785
2,743	2,821	2,901	2,983	3,068	3,155	3,244	3,336	3,431	3,529	3,629	3,732	3,838
2,791	2,870	2,950	3,033	3,118	3,206	3,296	3,388	3,483	3,581	3,682	3,785	3,891
2,841	2,920	3,001	3,084	3,169	3,257	3,348	3,441	3,536	3,634	3,735	3,839	3,945
2,891	2,970	3,052	3,135	3,221	3,310	3,401	3,494	3,590	3,688	3,790	3,894	4,000
2,942	3,022	3,104	3,188	3,274	3,363	3,454	3,548	3,644	3,743	3,845	3,949	4,056
2,994	3,074	3,157	3,241	3,328	3,417	3,509	3,603	3,700	3,799	3,901	4,005	4,113
3,047	3,128	3,210	3,295	3,383	3,472	3,565	3,659	3,756	3,855	3,958	4,063	4,170
3,101	3,182	3,265	3,351	3,438	3,528	3,621	3,716	3,813	3,913	4,015	4,120	4,228
3,155	3,237	3,321	3,407	3,495	3,585	3,678	3,773	3,871	3,971	4,074	4,179	4,287
3,211	3,293	3,377	3,464	3,552	3,643	3,736	3,832	3,930	4,030	4,133	4,239	4,347
3,268	3,350	3,435	3,522	3,611	3,702	3,795	3,891	3,989	4,090	4,193	4,299	4,408
3,326	3,409	3,494	3,581	3,670	3,761	3,855	3,951	4,050	4,151	4,254	4,361	4,469
3,384	3,468	3,553	3,641	3,738	3,822	3,916	4,013	4,111	4,213	4,316	4,423	4,532
3,444	3,528	3,614	3,701	3,791	3,884	3,978	4,075	4,174	4,275	4,379	4,486	4,595
3,505	3,589	3,675	3,763	3,854	3,946	4,041	4,138	4,237	4,339	4,443	4,550	4,659
3,567	3,651	3,738	3,826	3,917	4,010	4,105	4,202	4,302	4,404	4,508	4,615	4,724
3,630	3,715	3,802	3,890	3,981	4,074	4,170	4,267	4,367	4,469	4,573	4,680	4,790
3,694	3,779	3,866	3,956	4,047	4,140	4,236	4,333	4,433	4,536	4,640	4,747	4,857
3,759	3,845	3,932	4,022	4,113	4,207	4,303	4,400	4,501	4,603	4,708	4,815	4,924

Figure 13

The number of measurements taken and the mean length ± 2 S.D. of the ultrasound femur length from 14 weeks' gestation to term.

From O'Brien, G.D., Queenan, J.T.: Growth of the ultrasound femur length during normal pregnancy. Part I. Am. J. Obstet. Gynecol. 141:833, 1981.

Weeks Gestation	No. of Measurements	Arithmetic Mean (mm)	±2 S.D. (mm)
14	31	16.6	2.5
15	28	19.9	2.3
16	28	22.0	3.0
17	35	25.2	2.9
18	30	29.6	3.1
19	32	32.4	3.1
20	27	34.8	2.5
21	29	37.5	4.1
22	23	40.9	3.9
23	33	43.5	3.6
24	38	46.4	3.5
25	33	48.0	4.6
26	39	51.1	5.0
27	37	53.0	3.2
28	39	54.4	4.1
29	28	57.3	4.3
30	48	58.7	3.8
31	50	61.5	4.5
32	52	62.8	4.2
33	41	64.9	4.6
34	41	65.7	4.4
35	59	67.7	4.8
36	56	69.5	4.6
37	51	70.8	4.3
38	46	71.8	5.6
39	34	74.2	5.1
40	28	75.4	5.6

Figure 14

Gestational age as derived from the length of the long bones

From: Jeanty, P., Romero, R.: *Obstetrical Ultrasound*, McGraw-Hill, Baltimore, 1983.

No. of mm	Tibia Percentile			Femur Percentile			Ulna Percentile			Humerus Percentile		
	5	50	95	5	50	95	5	50	95	5	50	95
10	10+4	13+3	16+2	10+3	12+4	14+6	10+1	13+1	16+1	9+6	12+4	15+2
11	10+6	13+5	16+4	10+5	12+6	15+1	10+4	13+4	16+4	10+1	12+6	15+4
12	11+1	14+1	17	11	13+2	15+4	10+6	13+6	16+6	10+3	13+1	15+6
13	11+4	14+3	17+2	11+2	13+4	15+6	11+1	14+1	17+2	10+6	13+4	16+1
14	11+6	14+6	17+5	11+5	13+6	16+1	11+4	14+4	17+5	11+1	13+6	16+4
15	12+1	15+1	18	12	14+1	16+4	11+6	15	18	11+3	14+1	16+6
16	12+4	15+4	18+3	12+2	14+4	16+6	12+2	15+3	18+3	11+6	14+4	17+2
17	13	15+6	18+6	12+5	14+6	17+1	12+5	15+5	18+6	12+1	14+6	17+4
18	13+2	16+1	19+1	13	15+1	17+4	13+1	16+1	19+1	12+4	15+1	18
19	13+5	16+4	19+4	13+2	15+4	17+6	13+4	16+4	19+4	12+6	15+4	18+2
20	14+1	17	19+6	13+5	15+6	18+1	13+6	16+6	20	13+1	15+6	18+5
21	14+4	17+3	20+2	14	16+2	18+4	14+2	17+2	20+3	13+4	16+2	19+1
22	14+6	17+6	20+5	14+2	16+4	18+6	14+5	17+5	20+6	13+6	16+5	19+3
23	15+1	18+1	21+1	14+5	16+6	19+1	15+1	18+1	21+1	14+2	17+1	19+6
24	15+4	18+4	21+3	15	17+2	19+4	15+4	18+4	21+4	14+5	17+3	20+1
25	16	18+6	21+6	15+3	17+4	19+6	16	19	22+1	15+1	17+6	20+4
26	16+3	19+2	22+1	15+5	18	20+1	16+3	19+3	22+4	15+4	18+1	21
27	16+6	19+5	22+4	16+1	18+2	20+4	16+6	19+6	22+6	15+6	18+4	21+3
28	17+1	20+1	23	16+3	18+5	20+6	17+2	20+2	23+3	16+2	19	21+6
29	17+4	20+4	23+4	16+6	19	21+2	17+5	20+6	23+6	16+5	19+3	22+1
30	18+1	21	23+6	17+1	19+3	21+5	18+1	21+1	24+2	17+1	19+6	22+4
31	18+4	21+3	24+2	17+4	19+6	22	18+4	21+5	24+6	17+4	20+2	23
32	18+6	21+6	24+5	17+6	20+1	22+3	19+1	22+1	25+1	18	20+5	23+4
33	19+2	22+1	25+1	18+1	20+4	22+5	19+4	22+5	25+5	18+3	21+1	23+6
34	19+5	22+4	25+4	18+4	20+6	23+1	20+1	23+1	26+1	18+6	21+4	24+2
35	20+1	23+1	26	19	21+1	23+4	20+4	23+4	26+5	19+2	22	24+6
36	20+4	23+4	26+3	19+3	21+4	23+6	21+1	24+1	27+1	19+5	22+4	25+1
37	21	23+6	26+6	19+5	22	24+1	21+4	24+4	27+5	20+1	22+6	25+5
38	21+4	24+3	27+2	20+1	22+3	24+4	22+1	25+1	28+1	20+4	23+3	26+1
39	21+6	24+6	27+5	20+4	22+5	25	22+4	25+4	28+5	21+1	23+6	26+4
40	22+3	25+2	28+1	20+6	23+1	25+3	23+1	26+1	29+1	21+4	24+2	27+1
41	22+6	25+5	28+4	21+1	23+4	25+5	23+4	26+5	29+5	22	24+6	27+4
42	23+2	26+1	29+1	21+4	23+6	26+1	24+1	27+1	30+2	22+4	25+2	28
43	23+5	26+4	29+4	22	24+2	26+4	24+5	27+5	30+6	23	25+5	28+4
44	24+1	27+1	30	22+3	24+5	26+6	25+1	28+2	31+2	23+4	26+1	29
45	24+4	27+4	30+4	22+6	25	27+2	25+6	28+6	31+6	24	26+5	29+4
46	25+1	28	30+6	23+1	25+3	27+5	26+2	29+3	32+3	24+4	27+1	30
47	25+4	28+4	31+3	23+4	25+6	28+1	26+6	29+6	33	25	27+5	30+4
48	26+1	29	31+6	24	26+1	28+4	27+3	30+4	33+4	25+4	28+1	31
49	26+4	29+3	32+2	24+3	26+4	28+6	28	31+1	34+1	26	28+6	31+4
50	27	29+6	32+6	24+6	27	29+2	28+4	31+4	34+5	26+4	29+2	32
51	27+4	30+3	33+2	25+1	27+3	29+5	29+1	32+1	35+2	27+1	29+6	32+4
52	28	30+6	33+6	25+4	27+6	30+1	29+5	32+6	35+6	27+4	30+2	33+1
53	28+4	31+3	34+2	26	28+1	30+4	30+2	33+3	36+3	28+1	30+6	33+4
54	29	31+6	34+6	26+3	28+4	30+6	30+6	34	37	28+5	31+3	34+1
55	29+4	32+3	35+2	26+6	29+1	31+2	31+4	34+4	37+5	29+1	32	34+5
56	30	32+6	35+6	27+1	29+4	31+5	32+1	35+1	38+2	29+6	32+4	35+2
57	30+4	33+3	36+2	27+4	29+6	32+1	32+6	35+6	38+6	30+2	33+1	35+6
58	31	33+6	36+6	28+1	30+2	32+4	33+3	36+3	39+4	30+6	33+4	36+3
59	31+4	34+3	37+2	28+4	30+5	33	34	37+1	40+1	31+3	34+1	36+6
60	32	34+6	37+6	28+6	31+1	33+3	34+4	37+5	40+6	32	34+6	37+4
61	32+4	35+3	38+2	29+2	31+4	33+6	35+2	38+2	41+3	32+4	35+2	38+1
62	33	35+6	38+6	29+5	32	34+1	35+6	39	42	33+1	35+6	38+5
63	33+4	36+4	39+3	30+1	32+3	34+5	36+4	39+4	42+5	33+6	36+4	39+2
64	34+1	37	39+6	30+4	32+6	35+1	37+1	40+2	43+2	34+3	37+1	39+6
65	34+4	37+4	40+3	31	33+2	35+4	—			35	37+5	40+4
66	35+1	38	41	31+4	33+5	36	—			35+4	38+2	41+1
67	35+5	38+4	41+4	31+6	34+1	36+3	—			36+1	38+6	41+5
68	36+1	39+1	42	32+2	34+4	36+6	—			36+6	39+4	42+2
69	36+6	39+5	42+4	32+6	35	37+2	—			37+3	40+1	42+6
70	37+2	40+1	43+1	33+1	35+4	37+5	—			38	40+6	43+4
71	—			33+5	35+6	38+1						
72	—			34+1	36+3	38+4						
73	—			34+4	36+6	39+1						
74	—			35	37+2	39+4						
75	—			35+4	37+5	40						
76	—			35+6	38+1	40+3						
77	—			36+3	38+4	40+6						
78	—			36+6	39+1	41+2						
79	—			37+2	39+4	41+6						
80	—			37+6	40	42+2						

mm   Gestational age expressed in weeks + days

Figure 15

Mean fetal kidney circumference/abdominal circumference ratios and the standard deviations.

Adapted from Grannum, P.A.T., Bracken, M., Silverman, R., Hobbins, J.C.: Assessment of fetal kidney size in normal gestation by comparison of kidney circumference to abdominal circumference (KC/AC) ratio. Am. J. Obstet. Gynecol. 136:249, 1980.

	Gestational Age (weeks)					
	≤16 (n = 9)	17–20 (n = 18)	21–25 (n = 7)	26–30 (n = 11)	31–35 (n = 19)	36–40 (n = 25)
Mean	0.28	0.30	0.30	0.29	0.28	0.27
Standard deviation	0.02	0.03	0.02	0.02	0.03	0.04

Figure 16

Umbilical vein diameter in the amniotic fluid and liver in normal fetuses.

From DeVore, G.R., Mayden, K., Tortora, M., Berkowitz, R.L., Hobbins, J.C.: Dilation of the fetal umbilical vein in rhesus hemolytic anemia: A predictor of severe disease. Am. J. Obstet. Gynecol. 141:464–466, 1981.

	Weeks Gestation*									
	18–19	20–21	22–23	24–25	26–27	28–29	30–31	32–33	34–35	36–37
Amniotic fluid										
Mean (mm)	7.0	6.5	8.2	9.3	9.9	9.3	10.0	10.0	10.1	11.6
± 2 S.D.	0.8	0.7	1.0	1.0	1.0	0.9	1.0	1.0	1.1	1.2
Liver										
Mean (mm)	6.6	5.3	5.4	6.2	6.6	7.2	7.0	7.5	8.8	10.0
± 2 S.D.	0.8	0.6	0.6	0.7	0.7	0.8	0.8	0.8	1.0	1.1

* Weeks gestation was assigned by the biparietal diameter using the Yale nomogram in conjunction with the known last menstrual period.

Figure 17

Amniotic fluid alpha-fetoprotein at Yale-New Haven Hospital in apparently normal pregnancies.

1977–1979 (2-year data)				1978–1979 (last-year data)			
Weeks Gestation (Menstrual Age)	Number	Mean	Standard Deviation	Weeks Gestation (Menstrual Age)	Number	Mean	Standard Deviation
15	39	12.1	3.4	15	17	11.8	4.3
16	135	11.1	3.4	16	83	11.2	3.3
17	228	10.5	3.1	17	140	10.1	3.1
18	200	9.1	2.9	18	116	8.5	2.8
19	83	7.9	2.9	19	53	7.2	2.5
20	30	6.3	2.6	20	18	5.4	1.5
21	17	5.5	2.5	21	5	5.4	2.0

The above data were obtained in the Clinical Immunology Laboratory at Yale-New Haven Hospital with amniotic fluids from apparently normal pregnancies in the period June, 1977 to August, 1979. These amniotic fluids were free of fetal red blood cells.

Figure 18

Liley graph of ΔOD_{450} vs. gestational age.

From Frigoletto, F.D., Umanski, I.: Erythroblastosis fetalis: A basis for practice and prevention. In *Perinatal Medicine in Primary Practice*, J.B. Warshaw, J.C. Hobbins, eds. Addison Wesley, Menlo Park, CA, 1982.

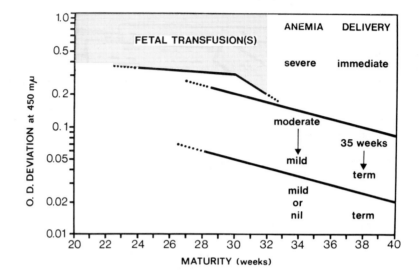

Index

Abdomen, fetal, 138
Abdominal circumference
    fetal development and, 92
    fetal weight determination, 71
    intrauterine growth retardation diagnosis, 103
Abdominal wall, abnormalities of, 140
Abortion, 18–20
AC: see Abdominal circumference
Adnexal masses, 28–31
AFP: see Alphafetoprotein
AGA: see Appropriate-for-gestational-age
Alphafetoprotein
    amniotic fluid, 127
    maternal serum, 126
Amniocentesis, 74, 75
    reasons for performing, 170
    Rh disease and, 82, 83
    second trimester, 171
        complications, 183
        management following, 187
        ultrasound and, 184
    third trimester, 188
        complications, 190
        lung maturity, fetal (L/S ratio), 188
        management following, 192
        Rh-negative patients, 193
Amniotic fluid
    analysis, 170
    blood taps and discolored fluid, 180
    diabetes effects, 77
A-mode scanning, 2
Amplitude modulation scanning, 2
Anencephaly, 121
Apple peel atresia of small bowel, 147
Appropriate-for-gestational-age, 87
Arrhythmias, fetal, 135
Articulated scanning, 4
Ascites, fetal, 147
Atretic valves, diabetes and, 80
Ausonics Octoson, 3
Automated water path scanner, 3

Bilobed placenta, 54
Biparietal diameter
    breech presentation, 63
    diabetes effects, 77
    fetal development, 92
    fetal skull, 34–44
    fetal weight determination, 71
    intrauterine growth retardation diagnosis, 97
Bladder, sagittal scan of, 14
B-mode scanning, 2
BPD: see Biparietal diameter
Brightness modulation scanning, 2

British Perinatal Mortality Survey, 90

Cervix, location, 49
Cesarean section, abnormal fetal presentation and, 62
Chemical compounds, fetal abnormalities and, 87
Chorion, 17
Corpus luteum cyst, 29
Cranium, fetal, 114–118
Crown-rump measurements, 77
Cystic fibrosis, 147
Cystic teratoma, 31

Decidual vein, entrance into placenta, 48
Delivery, ultrasound during, 72
Dermoid cysts, 31
Diabetes, perinatal mortality rate and, 76
Diaphragmatic hernia, fetal, 133
Dolichocephaly, 63
Drugs, fetal abnormalities and, 87

Ectopic pregnancy, 20–24
EDC: see Estimated date of confinement
EFM: see Electronic fetal monitoring
Electronic fetal monitoring, 205
Encephalocele, 123
Erythroblastosis fetalis, 81
Estimated date of confinement, 39
Estradiol, 214

Fertilization, in vitro, 214
Fetoscopy, 198
Fetus
    abdomen, 138, 140
    abnormalities, causes, 87
    abnormal presentation, 62
    activity, ultrasound evaluation of, 206
    anatomy, 113
    anomalies, diabetes and, 80
    assessment of development, 92
    blood sampling, 198
    breathing, ultrasound evaluation of, 203
    cardiac defects, diabetes and, 80
    growth patterns, 90
    kidney, 148
    limbs, 156
    lungs, 132
    radiation exposure, 194
    skull
        axial section, 41
        bipariteal diameter, 34–44
        corneal section, 41
    spine, 125
    thorax, 130

Fetus—*continued*
  7-week, 16
  8-week, 16
  weight
    diabetes effects, 79
    intrauterine growth retardation diagnosis, 102
    ultrasound measurements, 104
Follicle-stimulating hormone, 212
FSH: *see* Follicle-stimulating hormone

GASA: *see* Growth-adjusted sonar age
Gastrointestinal tract, obstruction, 146
Gastroschisis, 140
Genitourinary system, fetal, 148
Gestational age, estimation of, 34
Gestational sac, 14, 18, 19, 30
Great vessels, transposition of, diabetes and, 80
Growth-adjusted sonar age, 38

hCG: *see* Human chorionic gonadotropin
Head circumference, fetal development and, 92
Head-to-abdomen ratio, intrauterine growth retardation diagnosis, 98
Head-to-body ratio
  diabetes effec:s, 78
  intrauterine growth retardation and, 72
Head-to-chest ratio, intrauterine growth retardation diagnosis, 98
Heart
  fetal, 134
    structural abnormalities, 137
HMG: *see* Human menopausal gonadotropin
Human chorionic gonadotropin, 22, 23, 212
Human menopausal gonadotropin, 212
Hydatidiform mole, 25–28
Hydrocephaly, 118–121
Hydrops, non-immune, 144
Hypertension
  intrauterine growth retardation secondary to, 109
  pregnancy and, 84
Hypoplastic ventricles, diabetes and, 80

Infantile polycystic kidney disease, 152
Infertility, ultrasound monitoring, 214
Interventricular septal defects, diabetes and, 80
Intestinal aganglionosis, 147
Intrauterine device, pregnancy with, 31, 32
Intrauterine growth retardation, 46, 71
  appearance at birth, 88
  diagnosis of, 96
    integrated approach to, 106
  etiology, 87
  head-to-body ratio, 72
  management of, 108
  neonate, 88
  postpartum problems, 88
  secondary to hypertension, 109
Intrauterine transfusion, Rh-negative patients, 193
IUD: *see* Intrauterine device
IUGR: *see* Intrauterine growth retardation

Jejunal atresia, 147

Kidney, fetal, 148

Labor
  premature, 84
  ultrasound during, 72
Last menstrual period, dating of diabetic pregnancy, 76
Leiomyomata, multiple, 29, 30
Leopold abdominal maneuvers, 62
Limbs, fetal, 156
LMP: *see* Last menstrual period
Lung maturity, fetal, 188
Lungs, fetal, 132
Luteinizing hormone, 214

Measurement errors, sonography, 10
Mechanical short fluid path scanner, 5–7
Mechanical water path scanner, 5, 6
Meconium ileus, 147
Megacysticmicrocolon intestinal hypoperistalsis syndrome, 147
Meningoceles, 130
Meningomyoleceles, 130
Microcephaly, 122
M-mode scanning, 2
Multicystic kidney disease, 152
Multiple gestations
  amniocentesis,181
  diagnosis and development, 67
  ultrasound in, 69, 72

Neonate, intrauterine growth retardation, 88
Neural tube defects, 127
NTD: *see* Neural tube defects

Occipital-frontal diameter, breech presentation, 63
OFD: *see* Occipital-frontal diameter
Omphalocele, 143
Ovarian cysts, 28
Ovary
  morphometry monitoring, 213
  ultrasound evaluation, 210
Ovulation
  induction, 212
  ultrasound evaluation, 210
Ovum, blighted, 18

Perinatal mortality rate, diabetes and, 76
Phased focused linear sequenced array scanner, 5, 8, 9
Placenta
  appearance, 46
  basal or maternal aspect, 47
  decidual vein, 48
  diabetes effects, 79
  localization, 49
  morphology, 56–60
  second trimester anterior, 47
  umbilical vein, 48
  venous lakes, 49, 50
Placental abruption, 53

Placenta previa, 50–53
PNMR: *see* Perinatal mortality rate
Pregnancy
    diagnosis of, 13
    early, 13
        components of, 15
    ectopic, 20–24
    invasive procedures, 170
    ovarian morphometry monitoring, 213
    twin, 19
    with intrauterine device, 31, 32

Real-time scanners, 5
Real-time ultrasonic tomography, 3
Retroplacental clot, 54–56
Rh disease, 81
Rh-negative patients, amniocentesis, 193

SGA: *see* Small-for-gestational-age
Skeletal dysplasias, fetal, 158
Small-for-gestational-age, intrauterine growth re-
    tardation, 87
Spina bifida, 125
Spine, fetal, 125
Steered array scanner, 5, 9, 10

Therapy in utero, 200

Third trimester, complications, 62
Thorax, fetal, 130
TIUV: *see* Total intrauterine volume
Total intrauterine volume, 71
    fetal development and, 95
    intrauterine growth retardation diagnosis, 99
Twins: *see* Multiple gestation

Ultrasound
    definition, 1
    during delivery, 72
    fetal dynamics, 104, 203, 206
    infertility, 214
    labor, 72
    ovary, 210
    ovulation, 210
Umbilical vein, entrance into placenta, 48
UPJ: *see* Ureteropelvic junction
Ureteropelvic junction, obstruction, fetal, 152
Urine, production, fetal, 96
Uterine masses, 28
Uterine vein, entrance into placenta, 48
Uterus, midline sagittal section, 30

Venous lakes, 49, 50

X-ray, fetal abnormalities and, 87